The Armonk Diet

A Glutton's Guide to Losing Weight

Aaron Spingarn, MD

How to Eat All You Want and *Still* Lose Weight!

Printed in the United States of America

First Printing, 2017

ISBN 978-0-9986766-1-6

Knickerbocker Press
980 Broadway, Suite 542
Thornwood, NY 10594

Table of Contents

Chapter 1: Introduction

You really don't need a book to tell you how to lose weight. You can lose weight easily, if you want to. All you have to do is stop eating so much. It's so simple, anyone can do it! The hard part, of course, is dealing with all the annoying hunger and deprivation that accompanies your diet, because losing weight almost invariably results in you going hungry, or keeps you from foods you love, or both. Not eating causes physical pain and puts you through carbohydrate withdrawal. In addition, you don't get to experience meal satisfaction; and you resent not eating foods you enjoy. Losing weight mostly just leads to hunger and resentment, when it comes down to it. So you keep searching for a way that leads to less suffering. This explains why there are so many useless diet books and plans out there that want you to let them guide you through the process. But what if you could eat as much as you want, and mostly whatever you want, and still lose weight? Then weight loss would be easy, right?

Welcome to losing weight the easy way.

With any luck, this book will be the last weight loss guide you will ever need. If you want to slim down, regardless of your previous lack of dieting success, you can now take those extra pounds off for good. Are you ready? Good. But wait, there's more. You also get to eat all you want and still lose weight. And you will do it naturally, safely, with minimal effort, and all while completely satisfying your appetite. All you need is to keep an open mind and be willing to try something new.

The holy grail of weight loss is losing weight without suffering. It's all here in The Armonk Diet. How to eat all you want while still losing weight. How to not waste your hard-earned money on ineffective methods that don't really address the problem. How to avoid undergoing risky surgery or taking medications with unpleasant side effects. You will do this all by yourself, with just a little guidance from this book.

Before our current age of convenient and relatively inexpensive food availability, and before we learned about its health risks, obesity was encouraged because it signaled wealth and prestige. Some cultures and many people today still covet an ample belly. Football linemen and sumo wrestlers, for instance. But for most of the general population, not so much. Our society suffers from the scourge of an obesity epidemic, and has a very large overweight population, most of whom wish they could weigh less. But it's difficult to do. It takes a lot of effort to lose weight, and just as much or even more work to maintain that weight loss.

Why lose weight? Typical reasons include a desire for improved health, appearance, fitness, and mood. Losing weight reduces the physical stresses that cause wear and tear on your body's bones and joints. Your heart won't have to work as hard to keep your blood circulating. You may snore less and sleep better. If you have diabetes, losing weight offers your best chance of controlling your disease without having to rely on medication. Other medical conditions, such as metabolic syndrome, will also improve, and your risk of strokes, heart attacks, and some cancers will decrease. Additionally, you may want to look thinner in order to attain your ideal appearance, or to improve your prospects socially or professionally. Losing weight may improve your athletic performance, and could reduce the feelings of depression or low self-esteem that often accompany obesity. Most likely, you want to lose weight due to some combination of the above.

Ideally, to correct the problem of obesity, we need to change what and how we eat. This would involve addressing each affected individual's underlying reasons for overeating and then changing their ingrained lifelong poor eating habits through some kind of behavior modification - a project far beyond anything this book can offer. Practically speaking, most of us need a different approach, one that helps us deal with our weight issue now, in real time.

The well-publicized keys to losing weight are generally agreed to be eating less and exercising more. But putting those recommendations into action can prove difficult. Going from a plan that sounds good in theory to actual real-life results often leads to frustration and failure. You start out with the best intentions. But then, sooner or later, you get hungry, or you tire of the inherent calorie restrictions of most diets, and your hunger pangs take over. All of a sudden, your attempt to lose weight turns into an eating binge, and then you lose not only your battle for weight control, but probably some self-respect, too. Not surprisingly, among the numerous reasons why diets fail, not feeling satisfied after meals tops the list. Unfortunately, meal satiety (which is what researchers call how satisfied you feel from eating) usually requires eating more food than your diet permits, which defeats your diet. If only there was a way to control those pesky hunger pangs. Well, now there is.

The Armonk Diet eliminates the hunger pangs that sabotage your weight loss attempts. How? By keeping your appetite satisfied. Let's say, for instance, that you could eat something that fills you up without affecting your weight. Don't worry yet about what the something is. That's what the rest of the book is for. Just assume it can fill you up. So your hunger goes away. Without hunger driving your eating, with your appetite under control, you could choose to focus on eating only whatever you need to for nutrition purposes, or even for pleasure. You could choose to eat only the right foods for your health, the foods that you know your body will appreciate. Or you could choose to eat anything else you want, even junk foods if you must. But you could also choose to eat smaller portions because, with your stomach full, you won't be at the mercy of your hunger. With your appetite under control, you could consciously choose to reduce how much you eat. With your stomach full of the hypothetical *something*, you would lose your drive to eat, effortlessly allowing you to feel satisfied with less food than usual and thereby lowering your calorie consumption. The pounds would fall off easily. You could eat all you want and still lose weight.

The solution involves ignoring conventional weight loss advice. You do not have to eat less. In fact, you can stuff yourself to the point of bursting, if you want. You will control your food cravings by keeping your stomach as full as you need to, in order to ward off the hunger pangs that doom most diets.

4

The Armonk Diet relies on the magic of naturally-indigestible foods that fill you up. These foods occupy space in your stomach, but your body does not digest them, so you feel full without gaining any weight. Following this method, you can consume nearly-unlimited amounts of food if you want to. Here's why. All of your meals and snacks will begin with foods that fill up your stomach, which will make you feel full but not lead to gaining weight. Then, after you fill up, you can eat anything else you want for nutrition purposes or for pleasure. Once full, you won't want, or feel the need, to eat as much as usual, so you can choose to eat less. If you tend to eat until you feel ready to burst, your full stomach means you won't physically have the ability to consume your usual portions. So with virtually no special effort, you will start to lose weight. You can lose weight steadily, and you can keep it off forever, as long as you stick with this method. It sounds hard to believe, but it works. If you put in just a little effort, you can lose a substantial amount of weight. If you seriously desire a path to permanent weight loss, The Armonk Diet can help make it happen.

The concept behind The Armonk Diet, although simple-sounding and easy to follow, requires some flexibility regarding your eating practices. The Armonk Diet will teach you a new eating routine. Try to suspend your skepticism until you try it. Your diligence will determine your results. You will achieve the best possible results by following this method permanently. You don't need expensive ingredients, and you can buy everything you need at your local grocery store. Most importantly, you will not go hungry, and you will lose weight. Now you know the essence of the program.

Why should you listen to me? I realize that I am not a famous diet specialist and have not devoted my life and career to the careful study of weight loss. I'm just someone who wanted to lose weight and keep it off, like you. And when my previous attempts at dropping a few pounds met with long-term failure, I felt frustrated and wondered what made losing weight so difficult. But I ultimately conceived and executed a method to achieve my own personal weight loss goal and (surprise!) it worked. With this book, I am sharing this successful method with you.

In this book, you are going to learn everything you ever wanted to know, and probably some things that you didn't want to know, about gaining and losing weight. You will learn why you gain weight in the first place (hint: it's more complicated than you might think). You will learn about different weight loss methods, and why they do or (mostly) don't work. You will also learn an effective new method for weight loss that makes losing weight ridiculously simple and easy; and a detailed way to follow it, from A to Z. You will learn nutritional guidelines for eating healthily, as well as what vitamins and supplements you might want to add to your diet. If you need help getting started with meal preparation, I included some simple recipes to try.

The information in this book can help anyone who wants to lose weight, especially those who have previously struggled to lose weight and failed. In my case, for instance, I struggled with my weight all my life and, until I discovered this technique, found my attempts at losing weight too unpleasant to permit long term success. But now, over a year after starting The Armonk Diet, I am maintaining my weight loss without difficulty. The Armonk Diet can make the process of losing weight ridiculously easy. Regardless of whether you binge eat or just frequently eat smaller amounts, if you follow The Armonk Diet, you should expect to find success losing weight while still eating until you have had your fill.

Some disclaimers. If you binge eat frequently, you might have an eating disorder, which you should have professionally evaluated and treated by appropriate medical and/or mental health consultants. Also, you should not try to follow The Armonk Diet if you have any difficulty swallowing. You need to be able to swallow very efficiently and comfortably. In addition, I recommend that anyone already underweight, such as due to the eating disorders anorexia and bulimia, refrain from using The Armonk Diet method to lose even more weight. If you are not overweight by standard weight chart criteria, or if you suspect you have an eating disorder or want to determine if you have a medical condition that led to your weight problem, please consult with your doctor or another appropriate medical professional. Do not construe anything in this book as medical advice.

Why call it The Armonk Diet? Armonk, NY, is a quiet little hamlet in the Town of North Castle in New York City's northern suburbs best known for being home to IBM's headquarters and Frosty the Snowman. It also boasts a funny-sounding name that is easy to remember, and many of its inhabitants are amazingly thin, rich, healthy and gorgeous, providing an excellent inspiration for those hoping to lose weight.

This book is the product of a successful personal weight loss quest, and is intended as a guide to those seeking help in their own quest. It is not an academic treatise, and you will not find footnotes and references. What you will find is my understanding of current weight loss science, presented to you in a way that I hope makes sense. You will gain an understanding of why we gain weight, why it is so hard to lose weight, and how you can finally permanently solve your weight problem. Good luck!

Chapter 2: Our Relationship with Food

Glutton (glut' n) *noun.* One given habitually to greedy and voracious eating and drinking. Synonyms: binge eater, overeater.

In this chapter, we confess our dietary proclivities. Or at least *I* do. Not to seek absolution, more just to give context for why this book came about. Let's take a quiz! The statements below ask about your relationship to food. Give yourself a point for each statement that applies to you.

☑ People are amazed when they see how much food I can put away.

☑ If I see food, I generally want to eat it, hungry or not. I am on a "see-food" diet.

9

☒ I can pig out as well as, or better than, anyone else I know.

☐ I never leave food uneaten on my plate.

☒ No one ever had to tell me about how starving people elsewhere in the world would love to eat what I couldn't finish.

☐ Eating gives me greater pleasure than just about anything else.

☐ I find it difficult to limit how much I eat when I have access to seconds.

☐ My self-restraint for food evaporates once I start eating.

☐ I tend to eat until I feel too full, and often end up regretting not stopping sooner.

☐ It takes me longer than other people to recognize my body's fullness signals.

☐ I often think I could win in competitive eating contests.

If you answered yes to one or more of these questions, you may have some glutton in you. If you answered yes to all of them, welcome to my world, since I identify with all these statements, at least sometimes. Assuming you answered yes to at least one statement, no matter what your score on the quiz, your dysfunctional relationship to eating has unfortunate weight control repercussions. Sadly, it's not very easy to fix the dysfunction, but with the help of this book you can get it under control.

Okay, maybe this is a good place to confess that I was never severely overweight. At six feet tall and 187 pounds before I began The Armonk Diet, I barely cracked the overweight column on the usual weight charts. But I was never satisfied with my weight, and I had a number of weight-related ailments, including various musculoskeletal pains as well as snoring and obstructive sleep apnea. So I had a personal motivation to do something about my weight, even though my previous attempts at losing weight failed. You may be thinking to yourself that I wasn't overweight enough to really know the challenges of losing weight. And you may be right. But consider that my success in discovering how to lose weight effectively does not require me to have experienced obesity. If the method works, it works for dieters of any weight. Base your judgement on your results. I dropped 30 pounds following this diet. If you weigh more than me, you can lose more weight than I did. It doesn't matter how overweight you are. In order to succeed with The Armonk Diet, you just need to want to lose weight.

Consider my food issues in the context of your own dysfunctional relationship with food. Some people, most of whom probably don't have weight control issues, can stop eating before they completely stuff themselves. I am not one of those people. If you can regularly push away from the table without overstuffing yourself, then please accept my congratulations on your self-control. Personally, I find it hard to stop eating until my stomach feels ready to burst. So this is the context of my particular eating dysfunction. I don't actually snatch food away from others, at least not unless they offer, but my inner ravenous beast never seems far away. I eat too much food, mostly all at once, and often regret it afterwards. Yes, I am a glutton. If you are, too, then welcome to the club. In some religions, gluttony is a sin. For our purposes, there is nothing sinful about it. It is merely a problem that leads to gaining weight. It is not curable; rather, its consequences need to be managed. The Armonk Diet can help you get it under control.

We now move on to our relationship with meals. I have a history of maladaptive relationships with meals. Consider breakfast, for instance. From childhood through adulthood, I always woke up hungry, and not because I didn't eat enough the day before. If anything, I was too well fed. My parents stressed the then-current dogma regarding breakfast's importance as the most important meal of the day. I was informed that eating breakfast would give me the energy to start my day, and would help with weight control as well as improve my overall health. So I ate breakfast every day, usually cold cereal with milk.

But breakfast did not work out well for me, in retrospect. Sadly unrecognized by me or anyone else at the time, my lactose intolerance made cow's milk a poor intestinal choice to accompany my cereal, aside from the calcium it gave me. And the sugar in my breakfast cereals certainly gave me a morning boost, but the also-unrecognized post-sugar crash made me ravenous for more food well before lunchtime. So between the lactose in my milk and the sugar in my cereal, breakfast did not help me much. Not knowing any better, I stuck with my cereal and milk routine. Now fast forward a few decades. A review of the actual science regarding breakfast's importance in health and weight control refutes the old conclusions regarding breakfast's importance in your diet. No scientific justification exists for eating breakfast unless you want to.

Given a chance to do my childhood over (which really means what I recommend for those who are not dieting but want advice about breakfast cereal), I would recommend un-sugared cereals accompanied by water or soy milk. Helpful hint: it turns out that you can adjust very easily to water as the liquid of choice in your cereal bowl. (It just takes two weeks to get used to the transition.) I would have obtained my calcium some other way, such as from a supplement. Of course, if you are not lactose-intolerant, feel free to drink cow's milk, if you wish. As an adult, I switched to non-cereal foods such as eggs (egg whites, actually) and nuts for breakfast when I began following a low-carbohydrate diet. Eggs and nuts do not cause the same after-meal hunger due to their high protein, low-sugar content. However, I got tired of eggs eventually, and then couldn't look at them anymore. And nuts sometimes irritated my stomach, in addition to which their high calorie density does not promote weight loss. So much for breakfast. I now skip breakfast, aside from a cup of coffee, which I plan to continue until coffee starts giving me an upset stomach. I hope my stomach holds out. I now eat nuts with dinner for their health benefits, which we will further discuss in Chapter 15.

Now we come to lunch. As a child, I always ate lunch, because I was always hungry. I brown-bagged it to school, usually eating a sandwich with lunchmeats or peanut butter and jelly. Unknown to me at the time, carbohydrate-rich foods such as the bread in my sandwiches and the sugar in jelly can cause drowsiness about an hour after eating them. Thanks to my inadvertently-poor lunch choices, I usually had trouble staying awake in my after-lunch classes. The lunch-eating habit stayed with me all my life; so did falling asleep soon after lunch. Only when I stopped eating lunch did I stop nodding off in the middle of the day. Then came a post-carbohydrate crash in the early afternoon, which of course made me ravenous for a mid-afternoon snack. Between breakfast and lunch, my eating habits led to a lot of preventable weight struggles.

My gluttony really kicks in around dinner, my main and often only meal of the day. Dinner at home means I can keep eating for as long as I want, and I do. When I eat dinner with no one around to make me self-conscious, I can turn into a human vacuum cleaner. I feel myself getting full, but I just can't seem to stop until my stomach feels ready to burst. A more disciplined eater would stop earlier and patiently wait for the sensation of satiety to eventually arrive. I just don't seem to possess that patience. Even on The Armonk Diet, I recognize that my hunger pangs have diminished greatly about halfway through dinner but, if food remains available around me, I have this compelling need to continue eating until meal satisfaction sets in. Only then have I eaten enough. It can take me two hours to finish dinner.

If you can personally relate to any of the food-related dysfunction above, I feel your pain. We were given bad advice, because no one knew any better or, if they did, there was so much contradicting misinformation that it drowned out any good advice. And if you eat food in the quantities I do, for any number of reasons, you know you're not on a path to getting your weight under control.

So this brings us to my dieting experience before I discovered The Armonk Diet. For most of my life, I did no formal dieting, but just wished I could lose weight. This turned out not to be a good strategy. It seemed like I gained a pound or two every year, which I blamed on aging. The only diet I ever really tried was The Atkins Diet, which appealed to me because it allows you to eat all you want, except for severely restricting carbohydrates. I tried it, and it worked for me at the start, but I found the low-carbohydrate restriction too difficult to maintain. I did lose weight, and I felt and looked better. But carbohydrate deprivation eventually proved too difficult to sustain, and I eventually succumbed to temptation and gave up on the Atkins diet, and gradually the weight came back.

Here's what happened after I discovered The Armonk Diet. I lost about a pound per week for about 5 months. I had set a goal to reach 168 pounds, which I remember weighing during my school days 30 years ago. After I began following The Armonk Diet, I reached 168, and I realized I could keep going. So I set another goal for 5 pounds less, and then another 5 pounds. I actually lost thirty pounds in six months without changing anything else about my life. Since then, I have maintained my new weight without much of a struggle, including occasional cheat days. I am not going hungry and am still eating like a pig while following the simple diet rules described in this book.

Several changes occurred in my body after I started to follow The Armonk Diet. Let's start with the positive changes. I lost 3 inches off my waist size. My thighs used to rub against each other when I ran for exercise, which stopped after I lost weight, so no more chafing. My snoring and obstructive sleep apnea resolved, and I seem to require less sleep now. Various joint and muscle pains either resolved or improved with no other interventions. My wife, who used to kid me about my abdominal girth (she called it a muffin top), stopped. My veins stick out a lot more than they used to, which will be helpful when I want to donate blood. My blood chemistries were and remain excellent, with no abnormalities in my electrolytes, cholesterol, or in blood indicators of muscle, liver, and kidney function.

Now we get to the negatives of losing weight. Some in my family think I look too thin. Although I like my appearance, my cheeks do look a little hollow as my face lost some of its previous fullness. Some people who know me noticed this hollowness and expressed concern about my well-being. They thought I looked sick and asked if I was all right. Some made comments to my wife, asking similar questions. I am showing my age more; fewer people comment on how young I seem. Sitting down did not used to hurt, but for almost a year, sitting actually hurt my butt after a while, probably because I lost some fat padding there. The skin on my butt droops a little more than it used to. I have to exercise more to burn the same number of calories due to my lower weight.

So losing weight does have some downsides. But what a great problem to have! Would you trade a sore butt for losing 15% of your body weight? It seems like a pretty reasonable trade-off to me. Fortunately, the sitting-down discomfort improved slowly. And you could always correct some of the hollowness in your face with injectable fillers or implants. Although not cheap, fillers can be administered in a relatively simple in-office procedure.

You might reasonably wonder whether, as a glutton, I might consider trying to change my hard-wired tendency toward ravenous eating. Perhaps I might benefit from some kind of therapy to find and try to fix an underlying psychological reason for my eating patterns. Perhaps therapy *would* help. But I would rather just treat my weight directly, because I doubt that therapy, even if helps me identify a root cause, would actually fix whatever the problem is. And I don't feel a compelling need to spend my limited free time finding out.

I suspect that many eating disorders probably can't be fixed, because nature seems to conspire against losing weight. As you read the next chapter, you will learn how. And then you will learn how to get your weight under control by using nature's own tricks against it. You will see that every overweight situation does not necessarily stem from laziness or lack of self-control. Even if it does, with the help of The Armonk Diet, you can now do something about it.

Chapter 3: How Weight Control Works (or Doesn't)

Before continuing on to how and why The Armonk Diet works, it helps to understand how complicated your weight control process is. This chapter sets up the premise behind The Armonk Diet by discussing how and why we gain unwanted weight. This leads into what makes losing weight so difficult, and what makes keeping lost weight off so difficult, followed by what traditional weight loss remedies such as diets have to offer and why they often do not help. If you just want to get to the nuts and bolts of following The Armonk Diet, you can skip ahead to Chapter 8. But you should stick around to gain some insight into this complicated and interesting subject. You might be amazed that anyone could ever lose weight using only their own personal willpower. Once you see why traditional weight-loss remedies do not work very well in your personal war on weight, you might be more likely to accept The Armonk Diet's radical approach to losing weight.

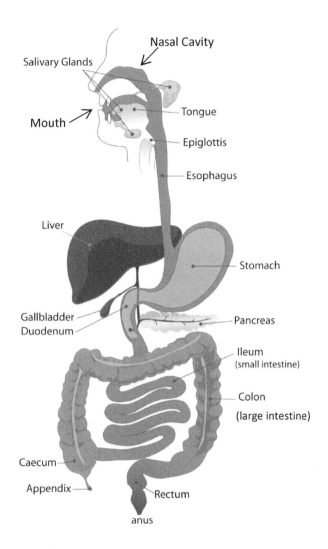

Figure. The Digestive Tract.

Calories

In any discussion about weight, you need to know something about calories. We measure the energy contained in food by referring to its calorie content. Calories, often abbreviated kcal if you read the science literature, bear a similarity to the kilowatt-hours of electricity that power your home. We define a calorie as the amount of energy required to raise the temperature of one milliliter of water (the amount of water found in a cube measuring one centimeter on each side) by one degree Celsius. For those not used to the metric system, it would take about nine calories to heat a cubic inch of water by one degree Fahrenheit.

How Your Body Processes Food

Let's take a brief detour to understand how your body processes food. Your gastro-intestinal tract unlocks food's energy. If you want to follow along with a drawing, take a look at the Figure. When you swallow food, it passes from your mouth into a swallowing tube, called the esophagus, which funnels the food down into your stomach. Your stomach serves as a kind of temporary holding tank. Food stops there for up to a few hours while your stomach grinds it up and mixes it with stomach acids. This results in your food becoming a slurry. The food slurry exits your stomach slowly, next passing into your small intestine, where most of the digestive action happens. In your small intestine, the food slurry encounters digestive enzymes, which help break down food particles into their smallest components, called nutrients, such as sugars (from starchy foods), fats (from fatty foods and oils), and amino acids (from protein). Your small intestine then transports these nutrients into your bloodstream so the rest of your body can use them. From your bloodstream, these nutrients can get to anywhere else your body needs them, such as in repairing muscle damage and replacing old worn-out cells. If the absorbed nutrients do not serve any immediate purpose, your body converts them to fat, which it stores all over your body as a reservoir for your future energy needs. This is where most of your excess weight goes. Non-digested food, such as fiber, remains in your intestines and continues on into your large intestines (the colon). Your colon compacts all the leftovers together as feces (also known as stool, excrement, and poop), slowly transporting it along until it reaches your rectum. Your rectum stores the feces until you defecate, which is commonly known as having a bowel movement.

Calorie Counting and Weight Loss Planning

Now, back to calories. Every nutrient (carbohydrate, fat, and protein) has a certain calorie density, meaning the number of calories contained in each gram of the nutrient. Carbohydrates such as sugar, and protein from sources such as meat, have 4 calories per gram. Fat, in contrast, has 9 calories per gram. Do you want to lose one pound of body fat? Although one pound of pure fat contains almost 4100 calories by the above calculations, body fat incorporates some other ingredients that reduce its calorie density to 3500 calories per pound. Want to lose that pound of fat in one week? That's 3500 calories divided by 7 days, which means you can lose a pound of fat per week if you reduce your calorie consumption by roughly 500 calories per day below what your body needs to maintain itself.

Everyone's calorie maintenance requirements will differ, depending on their age, weight, gender, and time spent daily doing various activities. If you diligently follow The Armonk Diet, you do not need to spend a lot of time thinking about calories. You can just follow the instructions and watch your weight drop. However, if you like structure in your diet program, you may wish to set a daily calorie intake goal so you can, for instance, try to consume 500 fewer calories than your body requires every day. This means you need to know how many calories your body needs to take in every day in order to maintain itself. You can estimate this number, known as your body's calorie maintenance requirement, by using a "total energy expenditure" calculator. You can easily find this type of calculator online, for instance at http://www.health-calc.com/diet/energy-expenditure-advanced. This type of calculator can tell you your Total Energy Expenditure, which means how many calories your body requires daily in order to maintain your weight. Just make sure that you check the "kcal" box, as kcal means calories, and check the "US" box in the Units section.

In case you wondered, you can't choose whether your body burns fat, carbohydrate, or protein. Your body automatically makes its own selection. If you have plenty of extra fat, though, then that's what your body will generally use for energy, with one notable exception. Your brain, differently from the rest of your body, relies on carbohydrates as its primary energy source. Your body does not store carbohydrates in very large quantities, so when your glucose stores run low, your body converts fat to glucose in a process called gluconeogenesis. Your body burns protein only when your fat stores run low, which we will discuss later when we get to starvation-type diets.

Why We Gain Weight

We gain weight when we consume more nutrients than our bodies need to meet our maintenance energy requirements. The amount of energy a body needs can vary for different people even when they weigh the same. This happens due to individual differences in the amount of energy burned. Some unlucky individuals may gain weight without seeming to overeat due to having a slow metabolism, also called a low metabolic rate. Common reasons for a slow metabolism include low activity levels, the effects of excessive stress and lack of sleep, high body fat percentage, heredity, and increasing age. A medical checkup can determine if you have a treatable medical condition that causes slow metabolism. Those of us without a slow metabolism typically overeat, commonly due to some combination of hunger hormone imbalances, emotional turmoil, boredom, genetics, expectations from family or cultural backgrounds to always finish the food on our plates, and the overall irresistibility of the prepared foods we encounter. Let's delve into a few of these.

The Food Science Industry is Partly to Blame

Most snack foods are inherently evil, from a weight-loss standpoint. You can lay some of the blame on the food science industry, the people who bring us junk food, for making it so easy for us to gain weight. Every snack food we eat has been conceived, focus-group tested, tweaked, and polished by food scientists who use every culinary trick they know to appeal to our senses and make us crave their creations. They know how much we love sugar and salt, and what textures feel best in our mouths, so they provide us with irresistible taste treats that do not exist in nature. As long as we buy their products, they stay in business to keep giving us more of the same. If we stuck to natural and unprocessed foods and avoided fast food restaurants, processed snack foods, and baked goods, a lot of us would overeat less and remain naturally thinner.

Some of Us May Have a Genetic Predisposition to Overeat

One hypothesis regarding gaining weight suggests that our genetic programming leads us to overeat to survive. DNA, the genetic code carried within all living cells and the result of many millennia of evolution, acts as a blueprint for our bodies and pre-determines everything from our appearance to much of our behavior. Some people, presumably for genetic reasons, do not feel full as quickly as others. They may have a condition called "fullness resistance," which makes them less likely to feel full after consuming an amount of food that would make others feel ready to burst. Those with fullness resistance have, from birth, a greater predisposition to gaining weight.

This tendency may have developed because, back in times of food scarcity, meaning most of human history, those who ate and gained more weight in times of plenty survived on their stored fat during lean times, whereas those without the genetic tendency to overeat would have starved during lean times, and so did not pass their genes to the next generation. The presumed genetic basis for this overeating trait thus survived by Darwinian natural selection, also known as survival of the fittest. The need to overeat no longer applies to modern humans living in a world of plenty, but hard-wired genetic tendencies can take generations or longer to go away. So we continue to overeat but no longer have a survival reason to do so.

The Psychology and Brain Chemistry of Comfort Foods

Comfort foods, whether mass-produced or made at home, often lead to gaining weight. Comfort foods predispose us to overeat by both satisfying hunger and triggering feelings of consolation and well-being. Research suggests that the

24

association of foods with happy memories affects us emotionally, impacting our perception of how good we think foods taste as well as how those foods make us feel. You may associate comfort foods with childhood or home cooking. Eating comfort foods often helps us cope with stress in the short term but adds to the long term issue of gaining weight. Common comfort foods include starchy items such as bakery goods, mashed potatoes, breads and pasta; sweetened cereals; sauced dishes such as gravy and chili; desserts such as ice cream and chocolate; greasy items such as chips, fried chicken, burgers, and hot dogs; and starchy cheesy fare such as grilled cheese, macaroni and cheese, and pizza. Although you probably realize that these foods stand in the way of a thinner you, and you may recognize the need to stop eating them in order to lose weight, the emotional component often stands in your way.

Brain chemistry probably explains why comfort foods provoke such strong reactions. This includes the activation of pleasure/reward circuits in your brain called neural pathways, as well as the effects of certain hormones on your brain and body. For some of us, eating demonstrates many of the hallmarks of an addiction. The relevant satiety-related neural pathways run on dopamine and serotonin, two chemical messengers in the brain known as neurotransmitters. When you eat something delicious, dopamine, a neurotransmitter associated with cravings, increases in your brain in the same way it does with drug addicts, new lovers, and attention-seekers. In addition, consuming carbohydrates results in increased serotonin levels. Serotonin helps you to relax, sleep, and cope with life. Carbohydrate-based comfort foods, then, seem particularly likely to drive continued food consumption even after you get full. You might conceivably try to gain control over this phenomenon by avoiding carbohydrates, as well as delicious foods in general.

Unfortunately, although medications can lower both dopamine and serotonin levels, taking these medications does not help as much as we would like with losing weight, and can cause unpleasant side effects, as you will see in Chapter 5.

An Abnormally Strong Hunger Drive

In many cases, gaining weight results from the inability to stop eating, even when you recognize that you have eaten enough. Researchers who study satiety report that normal individuals start recognizing that they feel full about 20 minutes after they start eating. The fullness sensation continues to increase for up to 30 more minutes. Stretch receptors in your stomach normally signal your brain when your stomach maximally stretches out, which helps you lose the desire to eat.

Stomachs can stretch a lot, by the way, frequently up to four times their normal size. If you try hard, you could probably consume a gallon of food pretty quickly. That's about 8 pounds of food. For perspective, nine Nathan's hot dogs weigh one pound. The buns for nine hot dogs also weigh about a pound. So you might expect that 36 hot dogs and buns would fill your stomach completely, if you have a normal-sized stomach. Interestingly, the world record for hot dog eating, 69 hot dogs and buns in 10 minutes, indicates that some stomachs can accommodate more than 15 pounds of food.

In contrast to those who experience early food satiety and have the self-control to stop eating before they get completely full, some overweight people don't seem to lose their desire to eat until well after they fill up. The desire to continue eating past the point of fullness suggests an either an abnormally strong hunger drive or a compulsion to eat. Science does not have all the answers yet as to how this happens, but a reasonable guess would be the presence of abnormally high levels of neurotransmitters in your brain's pleasure/reward circuits. High levels of dopamine and serotonin might conceivably overpower your desire to voluntarily stop eating when you approach satiety.

In addition to the neurotransmitters dopamine and serotonin, at least two hormones, ghrelin and insulin, may also affect your hunger drive. Ghrelin, a hunger hormone that signals increased hunger, also intensifies the rewarding pleasurable feeling that we get from food. Insulin can reduce your ghrelin levels, which reduces hunger. So from the standpoint of reining in out-of-control overeating, you might benefit from elevated insulin levels, which you could accomplish by eating glucose-containing carbohydrates. The resulting surge in insulin production might theoretically help suppress your hunger drive. Unfortunately, none of these strategies has yet proven very effective.

The Inertia of Eating

Sometimes, the problem is not due to genetics, hormones, and neurotransmitters, but can be traced to a simpler phenomenon, which I call the "inertia of eating." Inertia is a term from physics, and refers to the tendency of a body in motion to stay in motion unless an external force acts on it. Well, in this case, it's the tendency of your body, while eating, to continue eating until there is a force acting on it to stop. When eating, especially (but not only) if distractions such as reading or watching an electronic screen take your mind off your food, sometimes your feeding auto-pilot fails to turn off, even if your hunger has passed. Instead of eating to reduce hunger or obtain nutrition, it's as if mealtime changed into a fun recreational activity, and you just don't feel like stopping. The only thing that would alter the inertia of eating and convince you to stop is feeling physically ill from eating too much, or finding a different activity.

For anyone intimidated by (or not interested in) the minutiae of your body's weight regulation system, sorry about the science lesson. There won't be a test. The point was to demonstrate the complicated and hard-to-defeat reasons that make us tend to gain weight. The multitude of different factors that contribute to hunger highlights the futility of traditional weight loss measures. In the next two chapters, you will learn what remedies people often resort to in an effort to lose weight, despite having the odds stacked against them.

Chapter 4: Losing Weight the Usual Way

You already know that, to lose weight, your body must either consume less energy, or burn more energy, than it uses. You might reasonably conclude that your best chance of weight loss success relies, first, on effective dieting techniques, so you consume less energy; and second, on effective exercise regimens and "fat-burning" regimens such as supplements, so you burn more energy. Unfortunately, none of these techniques offers proven long term weight loss benefits. Let's see why.

In order to lose weight, researchers found, dieting gives you a better chance of success than any other non-surgical weight loss methods, such as exercise and supplements. Dieting for weight loss means you have to change what you eat and/or eat less. Most diets, in fact, demand unsustainable food sacrifices. You will probably have to cut out something you love to eat. This makes dieting difficult to start, due to our general reluctance to stop eating what we like. Some of us can tolerate this for a period of time, but for most of us the necessary self-discipline will not last long due to resentment of the dietary restrictions.

But with a weight loss goal in mind, you might just possess enough self-control and discipline to follow your diet for long enough to attain your objective. What happens once you reach your goal? If you resume your previous eating patterns, you will probably regain the lost weight. So can conventional diets help you succeed? In the short term, maybe. Unfortunately, the evidence suggests that most dieters aiming to achieve long term weight loss will not succeed.

Since eating less leads to your best chance at losing weight, this chapter focuses on the various strategies you could employ in order to eat less, whether by changing your eating patterns so that you feel satisfied with less food, or by following a restrictive diet.

Changing Eating Patterns

Changing your eating patterns means you stop eating earlier in your meal than usual. You then wait, and eventually your body's fullness signals should tell you that you have eaten enough. Unfortunately for many overeaters, it's not easy to stop and wait for satiety to set in. As we discussed in Chapter 3, fullness signals can take a long time to register. Meanwhile, once overeaters begin a meal, hunger cravings can overpower their conscious desire to stop early.

As an example of changing your eating patterns, you might try filling yourself up to a certain level of fullness that is less than complete, and then wait for your body to register its satiety. For instance, you could fill your stomach approximately one third of the way with food and one third of the way with liquid, and then leave the last third empty. Alternatively, you could just shoot for about 80% full, regardless of the proportions of solid and liquid. These methods require either lots of self-control, or some kind of internal fullness gauge for your stomach. Will you really stop before you are completely full? You might, if you possess extraordinary willpower. But anyone with that kind of willpower probably doesn't have much of a weight control problem in the first place.

Stretching out your meal's duration offers another simple (and potentially more practical) traditional weight loss strategy. This means eating slowly. As you learned, some people take an excessively long time to recognize satiety. Eating slowly gives your stomach time to fill up and signal your brain. By eating slowly, you can reduce how much food you consume between when your meal begins and when you finally lose your desire to eat. If you haven't tried it yet, eating slowly takes little effort other than paying attention to your eating process. Just put your utensil down briefly and take a sip of water between bites. Chew each bite until your food has completely melted into your mouth. Each of these tactics adds a little time to every bite in your meal, with the end result of achieving satiety after eating less food than you might normally expect. But mindful eating requires concentrating on every bite, which means no more multitasking while eating. And, if you start your meal feeling starved because you haven't eaten all day, good luck remembering to put your utensil down between bites when hunger cravings control your eating. At our hungriest, our eating utensil functions more as a conveyor belt than a fork or spoon. For those of us who eat on auto-pilot, trying to remember to put our utensil down and to keep chewing takes more mental effort than many of us are used to devoting when eating.

Diets

If you tried changing your eating pattern or used mindful eating techniques and failed, a traditional weight loss diet might help. Traditional diets often employ a gimmick, some quirky rule that sounds acceptable but limits or promotes specific foods to eat or a specific way of eating. Whatever the gimmick, it convinces you to tolerate the diet's other restrictions. Ultimately, any weight loss regimen needs to cut your calories to something lower than your customary intake.

I'm going to share with you a dirty little secret not usually admitted by the diet industry: weight loss diets don't usually succeed. At best, only 20% of overweight individuals will ever lose 10% of their body weight and keep it off after one year. Many researchers think the number of people able to permanently lose weight is more like 1%. Shocked by the dismal statistic? Don't expect the diet industry to tell you about their low success rate, since then you won't buy their products.

Maybe you have the idea that the composition of your diet matters more than the absolute number of calories you take in. The evidence suggests not. When it comes to weight loss, diets that restrict either fat or carbohydrates demonstrate no differences in their results. Ultimately, you can eat whatever you want when trying to lose weight, just with less total calories. Unfortunately, less calories means less food consumption, which is hard to tolerate over the long term. Your likelihood of accepting a calorie-restricting diet will wane over time, limiting your potential diet success.

Hoping against logic that a different diet gimmick might give them a better chance at weight loss success, many dieters eventually decide to follow an organized weight loss plan, such as those described in diet books. A bookstore's diet section can feature up to 250 different titles. Most of them offer weight loss plans, each slightly different from the others and all of them convinced of their own method's superiority. Some of these diets probably work well for at least some people at least some of the time, if you believe their testimonials. But most, if not all, don't work in the long run due to poor compliance on the part of the dieter. If you somehow (miraculously) manage to find a diet that works for you, and which you feel comfortable maintaining, you are a rare and lucky individual, and you should continue it. Use The Armonk Diet's methods to supplement your triumph.

For most of us, who have not found a perfect diet but want to know what diets we might try, the next sections discuss some common diets. You can choose from plenty of different diet methods. Some have stood the test of time, and others, the so-called fad diets, come and go.

Fad Diets

Fad diets often prove unhealthy, so you should avoid them. You will find most fad diets nearly impossible to follow for a long time, due to their restrictions. Think of them as either too dangerous or ineffective. Please don't try any of the following selected diet fads, some of which you may have heard of, as they either don't work or their severe calorie restrictions mean they cannot be followed safely for very long. I mention them mostly to condemn them.

- The Alkaline Diet claims without good evidence that your body functions best when its pH is higher than usual, and so does not permit acidic foods. It also bans healthy foods such as meat and dairy, can prove strict and complicated, and relies on complicated and potentially dangerous fasting regimens.

- The Baby Food Diet replaces breakfast and lunch with several jars of baby food, which each contain 20-100 calories, and then a low-calorie dinner. Following this method, you will probably go hungry, probably won't like what you eat, and probably won't be able to tolerate the diet for very long. If you do, you may experience nutritional imbalances and might consume too few calories for your body to operate at its best.

- The Blood Type Diet assumes that each blood type (A, B, AB, and O) represents a different evolutionary heritage. For instance, type O purportedly comes from hunter-gatherers, type A from farming societies, and type B from nomadic tribes. The theory states that you should consume foods consistent with your blood type's evolutionary past. So type O individuals would eat high amounts of animal protein; type A, vegetables; and type B, dairy.

- The Cabbage Soup Diet is a one-week plan that allows cabbage soup two to three times daily along with bananas and skim milk. Following this diet yields short term weight loss due to calorie restriction, and may result in burning off lean muscle rather than the hoped-for fat.

- Various Cookie Diets severely restrict calories during the day, advising you to eat a cookie or drink a shake every two hours or so (500 calories' worth during the day), and then have a low (500-700) calorie dinner. You will likely binge-eat at dinner if you try to follow this diet for any length of time.

- The Cotton Ball Diet uses a stomach-filling technique to curb your appetite. It has you fill up your stomach by consuming cotton balls soaked in orange juice. Cotton balls, although a natural product, do not constitute food and can cause intestinal blockages and lead to life-threatening complications.

- The Five Bite Diet allows you to eat anything you want, but only five bites of it per meal, with a maximum of twelve bites per day. This diet results in severe calorie restriction.

- The Grapefruit Diet starts every meal with half of a grapefruit followed by high-fat, low-carbohydrate foods such as bacon, eggs, and other meats. This calorie-restricting diet mainly functions as a quick fix program.

- The HCG Diet calorie-restricts you to two meals per day and requires the injection by a doctor of human chorionic gonadotropin, a pregnancy hormone. This diet brings you to the edge of starvation. There is no medical justification to administer HCG outside the realm of fertility treatment.

- The Master Cleanse/Lemonade Diet involves subsisting for days on lemon juice, maple syrup and cayenne pepper mixed in water. You can't help but lose weight while on the diet. Once you begin eating solid food again, the lost weight returns.

- The Raw Food Diet allows no cooked foods. Although healthy, it requires impractical amounts of food preparation time.

- The Sleeping Beauty Diet encourages you to stay asleep for days at a time, which basically starves you into losing weight.

- The Tapeworm Diet requires ingesting tapeworm eggs, which hatch in your intestines and cause you to lose weight until you subsequently take anti-worm medication. Besides the gross-out factor, tapeworms can make you sick.

- The Werewolf, or Lunar, Diet requires fasting at new-moon and full moon intervals. You will lose weight while you fast, but once you complete your fast, you are likely to binge eat, and the weight you lost will most likely come right back.

Popular Diets

Various popular diets include calorie restriction plans such as Weight Watchers, prepared food delivery services such as HMR, and extreme work-out plans such as The Biggest Loser. Let's take a peek at some of these.

Weight Watchers works well for many people. Weight Watchers assigns points to foods and gives you a certain point allotment per day. Some foods don't even count toward your point allotment. For instance, you can eat all you want of lots of different fruits and vegetables. The downside consists of tallying points for foods not on the zero-point list, the restrictions of foods you love, and the cost. Many Weight Watchers participants pay a monthly membership fee or a per-meeting fee for support. Weight Watchers tells you to listen to your hunger signals so you don't stuff yourself, which leaves open the possibility of feeling deprived. So, even though you can eat all you want of at least some foods under the Weight

Watchers program, you may find yourself not feeling completely satisfied after a meal or snack.

Prepared food services such as home-delivered meal replacement services take the hassle of meal preparation out of your hands, similar to the convenience of having a personal chef. They will package and deliver your meals and snacks in advance, so you do not have to think about your portion sizes. This could work well as long as you do not keep extra food around to snack on or to supplement your meals. But you will probably experience the temptation to eat more than your meal allowance, so you may fail to lose weight. When you eventually stop using the service, often because of the expense, you will most likely return to your usual eating habits. Since you did not learn new eating techniques to counter your old habits, you will probably gain weight again. The HMR Program, one prominent example, replaces your own meals with prepared meals and shakes delivered to your home. The limits on outside food choices may create resentment, leading to diet failure.

The Biggest Loser Diet involves following a healthier diet and lots of exercising. The recommended amounts of exercise may not fit well into your life. Don't worry too much about the expense, beyond buying the book, unless you travel to the Biggest Loser resort. You can eat any foods you wish, but excessive amounts of strenuous exertion can take a physical toll on your body.

The No White Foods Diet bars you from eating any foods that contain white-colored ingredients, which mostly refers to carbohydrates such as grains (whether intact in whole-grain form or as flour) and sugar. This means you can't eat baked goods made from wheat, corn (yes, corn counts despite its yellow hue), rice, potatoes, noodles and breads. You could make an exception for such nutritious white foods as egg whites, cauliflower, and white meats such as chicken and fish. Although simple in theory and quite effective, the No White Foods Diet requires a lot of discipline, and you might resent that you can't eat foods you love.

Some people interested in ultra-rapid weight loss might consider a "near-starvation" diet. Did you ever wonder how long you might survive under starvation conditions? Fun fact: a human being can survive for 8-21 days without food or water, and up to 2 months on only water. But just because you *can* survive for long periods of time without eating doesn't mean you should. Fasting can cause the most rapid kind of weight loss, but losing weight so quickly could lead to health-threatening and even life-threatening complications. Your body slips into starvation mode, which leads it to break down not only your stored body fat for energy, but also other tissues, such as muscle. Starvation fasting can cause malnutrition, dizziness, fainting, fatigue, and numerous other symptoms. Therefore, you should aim to eat a safe number of calories daily, regardless of your weight, to prevent such malnutrition-related health problems. Some medically supervised, very-low-calorie weight-loss programs contain as few as 500 calories daily, and often result in losing up to 5 pounds per week. This type of program should not continue for longer than 12 weeks. Once you resume your previous eating habits, you should not expect to maintain any short term weight loss accomplished using this method.

Athletes should pay particular attention to the effects of such rapid weight loss, which may lead to a reduction in their muscle mass, leading to impaired athletic performance. Participation in a structured resistance training program and sufficient protein intake can help reduce these losses. If you want to protect against muscle loss while you work on losing weight, make sure to increase your protein intake to, for instance, 35% of total calories, and to do resistance training in addition to any active-movement exercises. Resistance training includes weight lifting, squats, curls, planks, sit-ups, push-ups, and lunges.

A do-it-yourself dieter trying to lose weight without professional help should follow certain calorie intake rules for safety reasons. In any self-guided diet, due to the risks of malnutrition damage without the supervision of a medical professional, women should avoid consuming fewer than 1,200 calories daily. Men should avoid consuming fewer than 1,500 calories a day. Women who eat 1,200 calories and men who consume 1,500 calories a day will likely lose weight. To maintain current body weights, women often require 1,600 to 2,400 calories daily, while many men need 2000 to 3000 calories daily.

If you want to keep track of your calorie intake and compare it with what your body needs, you can calculate your body's approximate calorie requirements online at the energy expenditure calculator we mentioned earlier: http://www.health-calc.com/diet/energy-expenditure-advanced. To count and track your calories, you can weigh your food on a kitchen scale and look up its calorie content online at a calorie counting website or app. For prepared foods, you can check the calorie content on their nutrition labels.

For a safe way to lose weight without supervision following traditional diet techniques, reducing your calorie intake to 500 to 1,000 calories below your body's current daily calorie requirement (while keeping in mind the safe 1200-1600 calorie minimum discussed above) should help you achieve a 1-

to 2-pound weekly weight loss. You can accomplish this by filling yourself up on foods rich in fiber, protein, or both. Examples include lean poultry, seafood, fruits, vegetables, low-fat dairy foods, whole grains, soy products, legumes, nuts and seeds.

People who overcome the odds to succeed in losing weight, although few in number, tend to have some things in common. They keep close track of their weight. They also use portion control to limit the amount of food they eat, often by weighing and measuring their food. They tend to exercise frequently, put up with hunger, and resist cravings better than the rest of us. They find it easier to maintain a modest amount of weight-loss than those trying to keep off large amounts of weight. It's a lifelong project and requires constant attention. Staying trim requires more effort than most of us can expend.

Ultimately, no traditional weight loss diet comes without some kind of deprivation, due to the need to take in fewer calories than you burn. As long as you diligently follow your diet, you will lose weight. But you will only maintain your weight loss if you commit to following the diet forever. Realistically, a lifelong commitment to a diet that deprives you of something you love will probably not happen. You will see that The Armonk Diet offers you an alternative without the deprivation and restrictions seen in most other diets.

Chapter 5: Non-Diet Weight Loss Methods

Now we're going to take a look at some interesting alternatives to dieting that claim they can help you lose weight. These alternatives include exercise, dietary supplements, medications, surgery, psychology, making yourself vomit after meals, and stomach fillers. Many of these methods are either dangerous or ineffective and, apart from surgery, none offers much hope of success.

Exercise

Most self-appointed weight loss experts believe that losing weight requires exercising. Sadly, the evidence does not support this belief. Although exercise promotes good health and physical fitness, for weight loss purposes exercise counts for little. Exercise does lead to an increase in muscle mass, and larger muscles can help you burn off excess calories during vigorous cardiovascular exercise. So it makes sense that having more muscle mass might lead to burning more calories. But all that extra muscle does not burn many extra calories once you stop exercising. And your brain, which controls your hunger and cravings for food, tends to crave more calories after exercising, making it all-too-easy to inadvertently consume more calories than you burned with exercise. In other words, exercising could make you gain weight rather than lose it. Studies that use exercise alone to help people lose weight have generally failed to find any effect. Those fancy weight loss exercise regimens that you see on television? Follow them for fitness, if you want, but otherwise save your money and sore muscles, since they will probably not result in losing weight. Interestingly, and gratifyingly, exercise can be an excellent weight losing technique if you follow The Armonk Diet, which we will discuss further in Chapter 8.

Fitness Trackers

Did you think that a wearable activity tracker, such as a Fitbit, would help you increase your energy use and therefore help you lose weight? Fitness trackers help monitor your activity levels and indirectly measure calorie burning. The current popularity of fitness trackers comes, for many users, from their purported ability to help with weight loss by encouraging you to increase your activity level. Unfortunately, the available results have proven disappointing. A study showed that dieting adults wearing activity trackers for 18 months actually lost less weight than a similar group who did not wear a fitness tracker.

So why incorporate exercise into your life? Let's take a moment to discuss a few of the health benefits of exercise. The number one reason to exercise is to extend your life. Moderate exercise, including activities such as brisk walking, swimming, and mowing the lawn, for about an hour every day, lowers your chance of dying by almost 40% over a ten-year period, compared to non-exercisers. Vigorous exercise lowers your chance of dying even more. Even *some* exercise beats none at all. In addition, exercise helps your brain. Exercising, specifically running, increases brain volume, reduces the number and size of age-related holes in the brain, and encourages the formation of new nerve connections in the brain.

For purposes of fitness, you don't need to spend ridiculous amounts of time exercising to achieve fitness benefits. With a type of exercise called interval training, meaning you exert yourself as hard as possible for brief intervals of time, fitness improvements from just 60 seconds of working out can equal the benefits of 45 minutes of moderate exercise. So even if you have very little time to set aside for exercising, brief intervals of all-out exertion, for instance by running or using a stationary bike, can get you physically fit. It just won't help you lose weight. But try not to give yourself a heart attack in your zeal to get started with your new exercise regimen. If you are out of shape, you should discuss an exercise plan with your doctor and maybe a fitness trainer before you start.

Supplements

Walk into any health food store and look around. Notice that much of their business model depends on selling weight loss products. Unfortunately, similar to exercise, dietary weight loss supplements won't help you lose much weight, either. Despite slick marketing campaigns, no proof exists that dietary supplements can assist with losing weight. The US Food and Drug Administration (FDA), our protector of public health, has not approved any weight loss supplements. According to the National Institutes of Health's (NIH) fact sheet on dietary supplements for weight loss, which encompasses just about any consumable non-prescription product marketed for losing weight, nothing works very well. The NIH does mention that caffeine, green coffee bean extract, green tea and green tea extract, and white kidney bean *may* have modest effectiveness. But many weight loss supplements have potential side effects, some of them serious. The FDA has banned some weight loss supplements due to dangerous side effects. Don't jeopardize your health by trying unproven or unsafe supplements.

Non-Traditional Ways to Lose Weight

Now we come to some less-traditional ways to slim down. Like their more traditional brethren, these methods also purport to assist you in your effort to drop those excess pounds, so are worth knowing about. They include emptying your stomach soon after eating, training yourself to reduce food cravings, and preventing hunger by filling up your stomach with food-like substances or with a device.

Purging

Purging means making yourself vomit after eating. As unappealing and unpleasant as it sounds, purging can immediately reverse your calorie intake, but can also cause serious damage to your body. Purging is usually done by sticking your finger down your throat, and is mentioned only to be condemned. If you resort to this method to keep your weight under control, you may have bulimia, and should seek the advice of an eating disorder professional.

Psychological Intervention

As suggested by the classic theory of Pavlovian conditioning (ringing bells caused dogs to salivate on cue, in the original experiment), you could theoretically train yourself to reduce your hunger cravings. For instance, some dieters find that, if they wear a rubber band on their wrist and snap themselves with the rubber band when they crave food, it helps reduce their cravings. You could also try the higher-tech Pavlok. Pavlok, an electronic device also worn on the wrist, administers an electric shock when you snack or indulge in foods you want to avoid. The zap lasts only a fraction of a second, and you can choose the severity of the shock. With enough time for training yourself, the knowledge that eating something indulgent will result in a painful shock might help you subconsciously choose to avoid the offending behavior. Unfortunately, neither this nor any other craving-reduction method has been proven to help with losing weight.

Food-like Stomach Fillers

Food-like stomach fillers form gels in your stomach, which occupy space and fill up your stomach, supposedly leading you to feel full earlier than you would normally. They then pass through your intestines and leave your body via defecation. Anecdotal reports suggest that some of them help some people to lose weight. However, properly done weight loss studies have not shown any benefit, and they all have potential side effects. For instance, psyllium fiber, generally used for treatment of constipation, absorbs fluid in the stomach and expands, allowing you to feel full. However, psyllium fiber also causes an increase in defecation and can lead to dehydration if you do not drink enough water. Appesat, a tablet made from seaweed, expands in your stomach. It also has no proven effectiveness, may have side effects, and you have to remember to take it half an hour before a meal. Glucomannan, a fiber found in konjac root, which grows in eastern Asia, may help promote losing weight in some people, but a scientific study also did not prove it effective. You need to take glucomannan half an hour before a meal as well, and it can potentially lead to blockages in your throat or intestines. Stomach fillers are the closest weight loss equivalent to The Armonk Diet. Although it may sound reasonable to try out one of these stomach fillers, with The Armonk Diet you don't have to buy any special products or remember to take anything before your meal.

Stomach-Filling Device

A medical-device balloon could be inserted into your stomach and inflated to fill up your stomach. You swallow it like a pill which just happens to have a thin catheter attached, via which it inflates to balloon-size once it settles in your stomach. The catheter then detaches and the balloon stays in your stomach, where it occupies space. In theory, a stomach-filling balloon makes you feel full more rapidly than without it, because your stomach remains partly full all the time, and therefore has less room for food. Unfortunately, this device has not proved effective for losing weight, and also would not help a person who eats when not hungry.

Medications

Several prescription medications can potentially help you lose weight. None are recommended as a substitute for dieting. All of these drugs can rarely cause potentially serious side effects, and most are restricted to obese patients. Successful medication takers (many find medication ineffective or stop due to side effects) typically lose 5-10% of their body weight within one year.

- Orlistat (Xenical) prevents the intestinal absorption of fat in your food. Side effects can include gassiness and liver damage. You can obtain orlistat in prescription form, or you can buy it over-the-counter as "Alli."
- Bupropion/naltrexone (Contrave) probably affects your hypothalamus and the reward circuits in your brain. Side effects can include liver damage, seizures, suicidal thoughts, and possible heart risks.
- Liraglutide (Saxenda) promotes insulin production in your pancreas. Side effects can include nausea, vomiting, and constipation.

None of the above medications contain stimulants, which are regulated by the government as controlled substances. All of the medications below are controlled substances due to the presence of stimulants.

- Lorcaserin (Belviq) affects the serotonin receptors in your brain to promote feelings of fullness, which reduces your drive to eat as much as usual. Side effects can include drowsiness, headache, and constipation.
- Phentermine/topiramate (Qsymia) decreases appetite by its stimulant and central nervous system effects. Side effects can include birth defects and suicidal thoughts.
- Phentermine (Suprenza) works as an appetite suppressant on your central nervous system. Side effects can include mental changes and hallucinations.

Surgery

Surgery carries a tremendous appeal in its theoretical ability to fix your weight problem with a one-time treatment that continues to work for the rest of your life. The most effective operation reroutes your intestinal plumbing, but there are plenty of other options, some of which are quite clever.

One interesting option is to have a device surgically implanted in your abdominal wall that acts as a little escape hatch between your stomach and the outside. The escape hatch, called the AspireAssist, and created by the person who created the Segway motorized personal vehicle, fits into a surgically-created hole that connects your stomach to the skin of your abdomen, giving you a small trap door that you can open and close on demand. You can eat a meal, fill yourself up, and then go over to a sink, open up the little plastic trap door, and much of the meal you just ate will empty out into the sink, in the same way that water would drain out of a canteen that you turned upside down. You get much of the benefit of purging without having to make yourself vomit, but it comes with the disadvantages of requiring surgery and having a visible portal embedded in your abdominal wall. Now approved for use, this device led study subjects who used it for a year to lose an average of 30 pounds each.

As another option, you could undergo surgery to shrink your stomach so your stomach can't stretch as much. This results in your stomach not physically being able to accommodate large amounts of food without leading to vomiting. A common stomach-shrinking operation, the gastric band, squeezes your stomach by wrapping around it like a tight coat. Surgery can also permanently reduce your stomach's size by removing a portion of your stomach.

An intestinal bypass, on the other hand, disconnects your stomach from your small intestine, and reroutes that connection to lower down in your intestines. Recall from our discussion in Chapter 3 that digestion, and therefore most of your calorie intake, occurs in the small intestines. An intestinal bypass avoids much of that digestion, which helps with losing weight.

A newer procedure, an abdominal vagus nerve stimulator, sends electrical impulses from an implanted device into the nerve in your abdomen that sends fullness signals to your brain, in order to fool your brain into reducing its food cravings. Many vagal nerve stimulator recipients lose weight, but most do not lose as much as hoped. The theoretical benefit of the vagus nerve stimulator was that it is a lower risk procedure than an intestinal bypass operation.

Surgery often (but not always) leads to permanent weight loss. Unfortunately, there are risks to surgery. And, of course, if you dislike the results, you may not have the option to go back to the way you were. So for many prospective weight-losers, surgery seems too extreme. And even with surgery, you might not keep the weight off.

No matter what intervention you try in your attempt to lose weight, you might fail. Most of the time, you fail due to inadequate initial efforts at losing weight. You give up, or you just can't get started. But sometimes, something clicks, and you you manage to shed some excess weight. Congratulations if you achieved significant weight loss! Now what happens? Can you stop your diet, or your medication, or whatever other method you used, and expect to maintain your weight? Read on to find out. I think you already know the answer.

Chapter 6: It's Hard to Keep Lost Weight Off

If you somehow manage to overcome the myriad obstacles to initial weight loss and conquer your eating habits for long enough to lose your desired amount of weight, you have accomplished more than most people in your situation. Now you have a new challenge. Once you achieve your initial weight loss goal, you have to confront how to keep the excess weight off and prevent the common outcome of regaining some of, all of, or even more than, the weight you lost. The difficulty lies, first, in poor compliance with ongoing dietary restrictions and, second, in the ways your body works against you to regain lost weight. It turns out that our bodies subconsciously intend for most of us to lose the weight loss game even before we start playing. Here are some reasons why.

Difficulty Maintaining Diet Discipline

The start of any weight loss attempt typically involves a certain amount of focused effort, attention, and enthusiasm. But it's hard to maintain that initial level of dieting motivation. Your focus may wane once you achieve your weight loss goal, as may your drive to maintain dietary discipline. So you start to cheat. But it's a slippery slope that leads from little indiscretions to eventually completely abandoning a weight loss method that works for you. If you care only about achieving a certain weight goal temporarily, such as for a particular event (weddings and school reunions come to mind), you will probably ultimately regain the weight you lost, and possibly more. You might want to think about that before you undertake *any* temporary weight loss program.

Most weight loss programs lack eating pleasure, healthfulness, and/or practicality. Without these crucial elements in place, any dieter's willingness to continue the program will naturally fade over time. Realistically, most dieters dislike their diets so much that they can hardly wait to stop, because not eating what you like equates to minor constant torture. Although you could decide to continue following your diet forever, in practicality, most dieters choose not to.

Exercise Burns Less Fuel When You Lose Weight

Let's assume you are one of those dieters who successfully incorporate exercise into their weight loss regimen. As your body mass decreases from dieting, exercising burns less fuel. This happens because your fuel burn rate depends on your weight. You might burn 100 calories, for instance, if you run one mile in ten minutes while weighing 180 pounds. But if you drop to 160 pounds and run the same distance in the same time, you might only burn 90 calories. A lighter individual needs to burn less energy to complete the same task as a heavier individual. So, if you rely on exercise for a certain amount of calorie-burning, you will burn fewer calories than you used to, unless you choose to exercise longer or more intensely. This results in having to take more time out from your busy day to exercise, and increases your chance of injury. So unless you increase your workout, your calorie consumption will be less than it was.

Dysfunctional Hunger Regulation System

Suppose you do, in fact, succeed in losing weight and you have made peace with your need to follow your diet forever. You still face challenges as you encounter the long-term effects of disturbing your body's hunger regulation system. Your hunger regulation system determines how hungry you feel. It works automatically behind the scenes, so you cannot consciously control it. It defends your body against any kind of weight loss, no matter how much you desire to shed unwanted weight. This weight loss protection mechanism works against you to regain lost weight and can sabotage your best efforts. You have to battle an invisible enemy that uses several different strategies to defeat your efforts, including manipulating the hormone levels involved in hunger and metabolism; putting your body into the equivalent of hibernation mode; and an effect called metabolic compensation that might make you gain weight even when you diligently maintain your diet. Not only that, when you lose weight, food actually tastes better, courtesy of your brain's insidious trickery. All of these factors tend to oppose your efforts to lose weight.

Hormones

Hunger cravings come from, among other things, the combined effects of a multitude of chemicals traveling around in your bloodstream that tell your brain how hungry to feel. These chemicals, called hormones, travel to the hypothalamus part of your brain, where they create their effect. The hormones involved in hunger regulation include leptin and ghrelin.

Leptin comes from body fat, and signals fullness. So, if you have more body fat, you produce more leptin, which signals your brain that you do not need more food and helps keep your hunger under control. When you lose body fat, the amount of leptin in your blood decreases. Your brain detects the lower concentration of leptin, and interprets that signal, rightly or wrongly, to mean that you need more fuel. This leads to a desire to eat more, and counteracts your efforts to lose weight.

Ghrelin comes from your stomach, and stimulates hunger. Ghrelin levels increase with dieting and decrease after eating. Leptin and ghrelin act in opposition to one another.

Counterintuitively, leptin does not affect obese individuals as powerfully as it does the non-obese. This means that leptin will not reduce an obese person's hunger as easily, resulting in less satiety after meals, despite having plenty of body fat and leptin. Decreased leptin sensitivity among the obese, called leptin resistance, can prevent weight losers from maintaining their new weight for more than a few months. And decreased leptin sensitivity may not change for a long time.

Metabolism

Metabolism is the process of converting your body's stored energy into fuel. Like a car, your body needs fuel to keep going. Common fuels in your body include glucose and fat.

Glucose, a type of sugar, powers your brain. The rest of your body obtains most of its energy from burning fat.

Your metabolism determines whether you burn just the right amount of fuel, or too much or too little for your energy needs. The amount of fuel your body needs to maintain itself depends on your fat and muscle mass, as well as your age, gender, and activity level. A slow metabolism may play a role in hindering your efforts to keep weight off. Signs of a too-slow metabolism include feeling cold, stiffness, decreased sweating, weakness, and fatigue.

Your metabolism can naturally change in response to many factors, including losing weight. Losing weight causes your body to lose fat and muscle mass. Since you need less energy to maintain the remaining fat and muscle mass, your metabolism slows. If you consume the same amount of fuel after your metabolism slows, the unneeded extra fuel gets converted into fat and leads to weight gain.

Other factors can also affect your metabolism. For instance, chemicals from our modern toxic environment called persistent organic pollutants (POPs) can cause a slower metabolism. We inadvertently consume POPs in many of the foods we eat, from pesticides, and from breathing in polluted air, and our fat cells store them. POPs act like hormones and probably predispose us to obesity. As we lose fat from losing weight, POPs escape from our fat cells into our bloodstream to slow our metabolism even more, which can lead to gaining weight.

If you try to cut out too many calories too quickly in order to lose weight, your body will enter so-called hibernation mode, similar to a bear's long winter sleep or a computer's reduced power setting, and your metabolism will slow. This probably occurs due to the lower hormone levels of leptin in your bloodstream. Since leptin comes from body fat, less fat means less leptin, which ratchets down your metabolism. As you lose more weight and your fuel stores begin to run low, your power plant starts running more slowly, and you break down less fat for fuel in an effort to conserve energy.

The more weight you lose, the slower your metabolic power plant runs. This means that, as you lose weight, your body's calorie burn rate decreases even more than you would predict just from the amount of weight loss alone, making further weight loss increasingly difficult despite your low calorie intake and possibly your increased exercise. Frustratingly, this hibernation mode phenomenon means you will burn fewer calories as you lose weight than an identical non-dieter who weighs the same as you.

Trying to lose large amounts of weight quickly will backfire. Rapid weight loss makes your hunger regulation system react more dysfunctionally than slow weight loss. Therefore, when trying to lose weight, exercising patience will lead to your best results. Quick starvation diets can wreak havoc on your metabolism for much longer than just the time involved in losing the weight, thereby damaging your weight-loss efforts for the long term. The more slowly you lose weight, the more likely you will succeed in the long term.

Adaptive Thermogenesis/Metabolic Compensation

You learned above that you should expect a drop in the amount of fuel your body requires when you lose weight. In addition, you know that losing weight slows your metabolism more than you might otherwise expect. As if you did not have enough factors working against your efforts to lose weight, now you get to learn about the phenomenon of metabolic compensation, also called adaptive thermogenesis, yet another reason for a slower metabolism due to losing weight.

With metabolic compensation, your body burns even fewer calories than you might expect on the basis of weight reduction and hibernation mode alone, and occurs even if you take your time and lose weight slowly. This slowdown of your metabolism appears to arise from changes in your body's so-called metabolic thermostat, which regulates how fast or slow your body burns its fuel. The mechanisms for this include increased mitochondrial efficiency in your body's cells and complicated hormonal changes that result in decreased energy expenditure, decreased satiety and increased hunger.

Mitochondria, the power plants in each of your cells, burn glucose to generate the molecular energy used inside your cells. In metabolic compensation, your mitochondria appear to require fewer calories to produce the same amount of energy. This increased mitochondrial efficiency means that your body needs fewer calories to keep itself running. So, if you consume the same number of calories as always, since your body requires less than that to maintain itself due to increased mitochondrial efficiency, there will be extra leftover calories to get deposited as fat, and you will gain weight.

The hormonal alterations involve the hunger hormone, leptin; cortisol; and the thyroid gland and its hormones. As an example of how this works, a low blood level of leptin, which results from loss of fat, causes increased hunger and reduces thyroid function via its effect on your hypothalamus, a part of your brain that signals your thyroid gland. In turn, the resulting low thyroid function, called hypothyroidism, slows your metabolism. And cortisol, a hormone known to increase during stress, may play a role. Cortisol rises when you diet, leading to muscle breakdown as well as reducing the effect of leptin.

As a result of metabolic compensation, if you continue to lose weight, the speed at which your body burns calories, known as your metabolic rate, begins to drop, with an average decline of 300 calories per day in a dieter's fuel consumption. This means that an identical non-dieter who weighs the same as you (after you have lost a substantial amount of weight) can consume 300 calories per day more than you while you both maintain your weight. To take this example one step further, thanks to metabolic compensation, you could actually gain weight despite consuming fewer calories than an identical twin who is just starting to lose weight.

Remember how weight loss makes you burn fewer calories doing your usual exercise regimen, due to your lower body mass? Even if you walked around all day with extra weights on, enough to bring you back up to your before-dieting weight, metabolic compensation means you burn less energy exercising than you did before you lost weight. If you feel like banging your head against a wall in frustration due to the sneaky way your body tries to defeat your efforts when you try to lose weight (or because this physiology lesson is scrambling your brain), it is understandable.

Unfortunately, the metabolic slowdown seen in metabolic compensation can last for years, even after stopping active dieting. This helps explain why those who lose dramatic amounts of weight often do not succeed in keeping it off. For instance, after losing an average of 129 pounds each, participants on the television program "The Biggest Loser" burned about 500 calories less per day than other people their age and size. When the show began, the contestants had normal metabolisms, so they burned a normal number of calories for people of their weight. When the show ended, their metabolisms had slowed dramatically, and their thinner bodies unexpectedly could not burn enough calories to maintain their thinner sizes. Even when their weight increased, it turned out that the contestants' metabolisms never recovered back to their baselines. Their metabolisms remained slow, and the pounds kept piling on. Sadly, the contestants in The Biggest Loser program regained 70% of the weight that they lost on the show. In fact, after five years, almost half of dieters regain *more* weight than they lose, and dieters actually develop obesity more often than non-dieters.

The So-Called Set Point

Your body apparently prefers to keep you within a certain weight range. Obesity researchers found that, for adults who do not consciously try to gain or lose weight, their weight remains remarkably stable over time. Researchers believe that your body will naturally gravitate back to its "set point," a certain weight range that your body generally stays within. Your own unique set point varies depending on genes and life experience. If you try to drive your weight lower than your body's set point range, your body will resist your efforts and, if you successfully lose weight, your body will try to find a way to regain it.

Unfortunately, this phenomenon does not work in the other direction. Based on the preceding paragraph, you might think that the set point range means that your weight should naturally drop back down after you gain weight. It will not, most of us will find. You won't be surprised to learn that, due to an asymmetry in the weight regulation process, your body gains weight much more effectively than it loses weight. Apparently, nature's weight regulating tendencies can't match the overpowering weight-gaining effects of our abundant first-world diets.

You cannot control your set point. If your body's unknowable set point differs from your desired weight goal, you will struggle to reach that goal using conventional methods. Some researchers think that no one can actually lose weight outside their set point range, and that those who successfully lose weight long-term really just started higher than their set point, so they merely lost weight that they would have lost naturally in the first place. In other words, you cannot lose any more weight than your body unconsciously allows.

Now you know some of the many reasons why nearly all dieters fail to maintain their weight even when they initially achieve their desired initial weight loss. As a result, few dieters achieve permanent weight loss despite their good intentions and hard work. Based on the preceding information, you should not expect your body to participate willingly in your weight loss quest. Depressing news, right? It almost seems as if there is no point in even *trying* to lose weight. But hold onto that thought, because there is hope.

Chapter 7: The Solution

Based on the preceding information, you practically have to believe in magic to think you stand any reasonable chance of losing weight in the near term, let alone maintaining your lower weight over the long term. Assuming you use just about any of the weight loss methods that don't involve dangerous medications or risky surgery, your body will probably betray your efforts. Your choices almost boil down to either having surgery or giving up before you begin, due to dieters' dismal success rates. Even if you succeed for a while, losing weight requires a lifelong commitment, and failure will frequently lead you to end up heavier than when you started.

So you should not start a weight loss program without the proper motivation for the challenge ahead, a commitment to follow your plan for life, and an ideal weight loss plan. An ideal weight loss plan satisfies your hunger, allowing you to maintain your weight loss forever without feeling deprived; and integrates seamlessly into your life so you don't have to obsess over the details or even really think about it much. Conventional weight loss plans do not fulfill these criteria.

Consider, instead, a different way, The Armonk Diet. You will not need an operation or have to take medication. You will lose weight by losing your desire to eat, which will happen when you fill up your stomach in a way that does not contribute to gaining weight. The Armonk Diet allows you to achieve and maintain weight loss while eating what you like (within reason), avoiding hunger, and not feeling deprived. This makes it easy to maintain dietary self-control. You can control how fast or slow you lose weight, although we learned that you will achieve the best long term results by proceeding slowly. The ease of following this technique means that you will not mind staying on The Armonk Diet in order to maintain your improvement. You will not have to stop eating regular healthy food in whatever quantities you desire. And even if you eat out of stress, habit or boredom rather than hunger, you can still lose weight following this method. You can lose almost any amount of weight following this method. However, you should discuss a healthy weight goal with your doctor before you get started, so that you don't drop into an unhealthy weight range.

The Armonk Diet can't do anything to fix whatever underlying factors led you to gain weight. But following The Armonk Diet can help you bypass those issues by lowering your hunger. This gives you the opportunity to choose to eat less, thus reducing your calorie consumption. The Armonk Diet allows you to experience fullness before you arrive at the point in your meal when you start eating anything that counts against your weight. By ultimately reducing the amount of food you eat, you will get your weight under control. In the next chapter we will discuss how The Armonk Diet pairs an effective weight loss regimen with dietary satisfaction to achieve long term weight loss, allowing you to join the rarified ranks of dieters able to achieve permanent weight loss without going through all the unpleasantness of traditional weight loss methods.

You can't beat nature with willpower alone. You have to outwit nature by taking advantage of nature's own tools. The Armonk Diet is the dieting equivalent of methadone for a heroin addiction. As with methadone, you never cure the addiction, but you can keep it under control and get healthier. Unlike with methadone, you do not need a doctor's involvement and you can do it all on your own.

The next chapter sets the stage to do just that.

Chapter 8: The Theory behind The Armonk Diet

We gain weight because we eat too much relative to our body's energy needs. Hunger drives our desire to eat. But what if you could remove hunger from the equation so that you no longer experience severe food cravings or hunger pangs? You might then choose to eat mostly to live, rather than live to eat. You might eat only for nutrition purposes, and you could decide to consume only the healthiest foods for your body, in appropriately small quantities.

You might still choose to eat for pleasure or socialization, or for other reasons not related to hunger. But once you separate hunger from your food choices, you have the power to choose to eat less. When you eat less than your body requires for maintenance of your current weight, you lose weight, regardless of all the tricks you just learned that your body uses to try to get you to regain what you lost. Taking hunger out of the picture can jump-start your journey to weight loss.

Spoiling your Appetite

Restaurants know that their patrons like to nibble on something while they await their order. So a waiter will often bring a bread basket or something similar to the table after you order. So imagine that you are hungry and sitting in a restaurant with a bread basket in front of you. Can you hear it calling to you? Can you also hear your inner voice telling you not to fill up on the bread because it will spoil your appetite? If you fill up on the bread, you might not want to eat the food you just ordered. That would be a waste, right?

The Armonk Diet turns the tables completely. Except that it's not an actual bread basket that fills you up. Call it a hypothetical bread basket. You *want* to fill up on the hypothetical bread basket because you *want* to spoil your appetite before the food comes. Why? Because your food contains calories, and your hypothetical "bread basket" is calorie-free. Your spoiled appetite means you won't need to eat as much. You will fill up your stomach with hypothetical bread and lose some or all of your appetite before eating the food part of your meal that counts for nutrition or pleasure and adds calories.

The Armonk Diet offers a practical way to fill you up and spoil your appetite. You will lose your drive to eat, which helps you shed pounds.

Remember all those diets that restrict your portion sizes to cut down on calories? They make you stop eating after you have finished their designated unsatisfying portion of food. You can now ignore the portion-size restrictions of other diet plans. Instead, you can decide to stop eating whenever you feel full enough and do not feel a need to eat any more.

You will not have to buy expensive proprietary meal products, follow restrictive programs, or experience any inconvenience. You will fill your stomach with natural food. It will not leave your body by draining out of a stomach porthole into a sink, or by purging. Instead, you will learn how to consume natural foods in a way that makes them calorie-free. This food will fill you up and will then pass through your intestinal tract naturally, without undergoing digestion, until it exits your body in the usual way. Your stomach will continue to feel full for at least as long as it normally would after eating any meal.

Don't worry if you eat slowly, or if it takes a long time for you to experience fullness. It won't matter how long it normally takes you to feel full, if you spend that time filling yourself up non-calorically. You should expect to lose weight easily because, once you have filled up, the next-up, calorie-containing, portion of your meal will not tempt you as much as usual, reducing your desire to eat as much as usual, so you will hopefully choose to eat less than usual.

Although your meals will contain as much food as you need to eat to get full, your eating routine will flow differently. Specifically, you will divide your meals. Think of your meals as split into two courses: the "bread basket" course, during which you will spoil your appetite, which we will call the *first course*; and the food you eat afterwards for nutrition or pleasure purposes, which we will call the *second course*. During the first course, the "bread basket" part, you will fill up on foods that do not count toward gaining weight.

Let's talk about how you will consume your first course. Dictionaries generally define "eating" as putting food in your mouth, chewing it, and then swallowing it. Your first course foods contain calories just like any other foods, but you will not "eat" them in the conventional way. These first course foods have an indigestible covering which, when swallowed without chewing, prevents digestion and renders them invisible to your body from the standpoint of nutrient absorption. In other words, you can swallow unlimited amounts of these foods, and no digestion will occur, no calories will be absorbed, and you will not gain weight. So you will not "eat" the first part of your meal, at least not per the definition of eating that involves chewing. Rather, instead of chewing the food in your first course, you will swallow it without chewing. Since your body does not digest this food, the calories in your first course will not count against you. Your stomach will fill up just as much as with any equal amount of conventionally-eaten food, which will efficiently ease your hunger.

To restate the main point of this discussion, no matter how much first-course food you swallow, you will not gain weight from it. Yes, the swallowed food weighs a certain amount, and yes, it will remain inside your body as it passes through your intestines. Therefore, you will temporarily weigh a little more until it finally comes out the other end, but you will not absorb any calories from it and you will not gain an ounce of extra weight as a result. In the meantime, your hunger will diminish because your appetite doesn't know or care whether you chewed your food or not. A pound of food will fill you up just as much whether you swallow it chewed or unchewed. As you fill up on food that contributes no calories to your body, you will eventually lose your drive to keep eating. Remember how overweight people may experience fullness resistance?

Following The Armonk Diet means you can spend as long as it takes to swallow as much first-course food as necessary to fill you up.

Will you experience eating pleasure from swallowing all that food during your first course? Probably not at first. But you will fill up. And if you need it, Chapter 12 will describe ways to make your first course foods more palatable. After your first course, once you have reached sufficient fullness, you then move on to the second course, during which you can eat what you like for nutrition or pleasure. The only calories you absorb, eating pleasure you experience, and whatever potential weight you gain, will come from what you eat during your second course.

Which Calories Count

Let's take a step back for a moment. To determine whether or not you lose weight, the number of calories in the food you swallow does not actually matter, because not all calories lead to gaining weight. Calories only count toward gaining weight if your body can absorb them. Calories only get absorbed from *digestible* food. The Armonk Diet relies on consuming *indigestible* food.

Here's a way to think about how The Armonk Diet works. As a thought experiment, and please don't try this at home, consider what might happen if you ate your favorite treat, perhaps a doughnut, but first sealed it in a plastic sandwich bag. Imagine that you then put the plastic-sealed doughnut in your mouth and could successfully swallow it whole. Of course, you shouldn't actually swallow a plastic bag but, for the sake of this thought experiment, assume that you did. You would not find the plastic taste of this snack very satisfying, but you would have succeeded in swallowing your doughnut. Did you gain any weight from the doughnut? No, because your body cannot digest plastic, so the calories contained inside the bag, wherein resided your doughnut, never get digested or absorbed. Eventually, the bag passes through your intestines and comes out unchanged in a bowel movement. So despite swallowing your favorite treat, and all the calories that came with it, you would gain no weight due to its plastic shielding.

You could swallow all the treats that you want in this way, enough to fill you up so much that you have no further desire to eat. Your stomach cannot tell that you tricked it by filling it up with something indigestible. Your taste buds, teeth and brain would know, but your stomach only knows that something filled it up. More importantly, your stomach determines your satiety, since your stomach sends fullness signals to your brain. Your drive to eat thus diminishes, without consuming any absorbed calories.

The more you eat of these hypothetically indigestible calories, the more you fill up, and the less you will feel the drive to eat regular (digestible) food with its absorbable calories. That's what your first course does. From eating less second-course food, you either gained less weight than you would have, or you experienced a net weight loss. In fact, the larger the indigestible first-course portion of your meal, and the more full you get, the less second-course food you will eat and the more weight you will lose. You can stuff your face and lose weight! Why? As the result of your first course filling you up with non-absorbed calories, you eat less second course food, which leads to less absorbed calories, so you lose weight.

You don't have to swallow plastic bags of food to accomplish this goal. Several perfectly normal foods will resist digestion if you swallow them whole. Specifically, you can rely on something safe, cheap, and easy-to-find in many different varieties: seeds. Seeds, as plant products, often have indigestible, impermeable outer coverings called seed coats. Seed coats protect seeds from external forces. Unless something penetrates or disrupts a seed coat, the seed within stays dormant and will not germinate into a plant. Humans *cannot digest* seed coats. Your body's digestive process cannot penetrate that covering unless you break it apart mechanically by chewing or otherwise destroying the integrity of the seed coat during food preparation or consumption. The calories contained inside seeds with intact seed coats are therefore also indigestible. Nature handed us a way to lose weight and defeat your body's sneaky attempts to fight against your efforts.

Lots of other natural substances cannot be digested and therefore contain indigestible calories, such as grass, leaves, and tree bark. But that's not food, and would not be tolerable to swallow or would endanger your intestinal health if you did. You can consume seeds, on the other hand, just like you consume any other foods.

In order for The Armonk Diet to work, *you have to swallow the seeds whole.* Intact seed coats are nature's equivalent of sealing your food in a plastic bag. You should not chew the seed part of your meal, or else this method will not work. If you swallow enough seeds whole, without chewing, you almost can't help but lose weight. None of the calories contained inside the seeds that you swallow unchewed will undergo digestion because your body's digestive process cannot get to them. But your stomach will fill up and your hunger will pass.

As long as you swallow seeds with intact seed coats as your first course, those seeds will pass unchanged all the way through your intestinal tract. You will start every meal swallowing as large a portion of seeds as you choose. You will fill yourself up and satisfy your hunger cravings before you even get to your second course. You will then eat your second course, chewing your food in the usual way for nutrition or pleasure. Hopefully, once you feel full enough from your first course, you will feel less of a drive to eat during your second course. If all goes as planned, you almost can't help eating less than usual during your second course, thereby reducing your total calorie intake, and allowing you to lose weight.

About Seeds

Not all seeds will work equally well for this task. You want seeds soft enough to swallow comfortably and that will not break apart during the swallowing and digestion processes. Two seed varieties, whole kernels of corn as well as beans, fulfill these criteria. Of these two seed types, you will find whole kernels of corn the easiest way to start this diet, due to their ease of swallowing and preparation. Other types of seeds do not work as well with The Armonk Diet. I do not recommend hard seeds, such as nuts and sunflower seeds, which will cause throat discomfort when swallowed whole. I also do not recommend soft mushy seeds such as cooked peas, because swallowing them tends to result in breaking their seed coat, which renders them digestible and defeats the calorie-shielding purpose of the first course.

Broken seed coats potentially present a problem. You will see this in beans mangled during the picking process, and in well-cooked beans, but not so much with whole kernel corn. Once seed coats lose their integrity, as with cooked beans that have a disrupted seed coat, your intestines may digest them in the same way as regular food. Interestingly, with uncooked beans, broken seed coats may not make as much of a difference, as whole swallowed uncooked beans appear to resist digestion, even with absent seed coats.

You might wonder, after closely inspecting some whole corn kernels, if they might be digestible. You might notice that the base of the corn kernel has an opening where the kernel formerly attached to its cob. The opening at the base of the kernel occurs as an unavoidable part of processing when a machine shears the kernel from the cob. You might assume that your body's digestive enzymes would enter that little opening and lead to digesting the interior of the kernel, which would affect the results of your diet. Fortunately, this does not seem to occur. All the whole corn kernels you swallow seem to exit your body looking pretty much like they did when they entered. Something about whole corn kernels makes them impervious to your body's digestive system despite that small opening along the base.

To summarize, certain seeds such as whole kernels of corn and intact beans have a seed coat that resists digestion. If you swallow these seeds without chewing them, you can fill up on them. Your stomach, which determines your fullness, cannot tell the difference between food you chew and food you swallow whole. The more you fill yourself up during a first course with seeds that have intact seed coats, the less hunger drive you will have for whatever food comprises your second course. This gives you the opportunity to reduce your overall calorie consumption and lose weight. The Armonk Diet does not depend on exercising, joining a support group, or buying prepared meals. Your meals will now have two distinct parts, with eating for nutrition or pleasure at the end. You can choose a specific amount of food to eat in advance, or you can decide spur-of-the-moment after your first course how much more you want to eat. You can eat all you want, and even stuff yourself if desired, and still lose weight, as long as you first fill yourself up on swallowed seeds before you get to your meal's second course. If you still have a decent appetite left when you begin your second course, this just means that you need to consume a larger first course. Just go back and continue your first course eating until you feel full, then remember how much it took to fill you up when the time comes for your next meal.

It might interest you to know how many calories you save when you swallow whole corn kernels and intact beans. A 15-ounce can of corn contains about 280 calories, if you eat it in the usual manner. A similarly-sized can of beans contains about 315 calories. So, if you eat three cans of corn and two cans of beans the usual way, rather than following The Armonk Diet method, you will consume almost 1500 calories. Following The Armonk Diet will save you those 1500 calories and fill you up just as much.

If You Overeat for Reasons besides Hunger

For those who eat out of habit, boredom, stress, or for any reason besides hunger, or who have an insatiable appetite and just never really feel full, The Armonk Diet may still work for you. When you want to eat, just follow the instructions for first-course eating, and you will probably lose weight no matter how much you eat. Save second-course eating for only designated times of the day when you need the nutrition. If you find that you cannot lose weight following The Armonk Diet, it probably means you need to take a look at what you consumed during your second courses to see if you have exceeded your body's energy requirements. Remember, you need to fill up during your first course in order to reduce the calorie consumption of the second course. If that means stuffing yourself completely by swallowing whole kernels of corn, then that's what you need to do. As long as you reduce your day's second-course calories to below your body's calorie requirements, you can swallow all the seeds you want, as often as you want, and your excess weight will fall off.

Some Additional Thoughts

With The Armonk Diet, you don't have to constantly obsess about food. Unless you want to, you do not have to weigh or measure portion sizes or count calories. You simply begin every meal or snack by filling yourself up on food that does not contribute to your weight and, once full, you can eat whatever else you want for nutrition and pleasure purposes. Just don't leave so much room in your stomach that you feel the need to overdo your second course.

Once you get the hang of it, it becomes automatic. If you follow a daily meal routine, it requires even less effort. You can snack all you want between meals, too. Just stick to the rules. You can abide by The Armonk Diet as a stand-alone do-it-yourself method, or do it in conjunction with any other diet method. It's your choice.

If you want to deliberately defeat The Armonk Diet, of course, you will probably succeed. Although you can eat anything you like for your second course, for instance, you can't actually eat unlimited amounts of whatever high calorie junk you want during your second course and expect to lose much weight. You should plan on making reasonable choices for your second course. A bag of potato chips and a box of chocolates will not lead to a good outcome. You have to take this seriously in order for it to work. Consider selecting healthier, less-appetizing foods for your second course to give you better results than if you choose delicious junk and comfort foods.

You can also fail on The Armonk Diet if you force yourself to eat past the point of satiety. So try to stop eating when you feel full enough. But you don't have to stop if you are still hungry, unlike most other diets.

You *can* lose weight while consuming virtually unlimited amounts of first course foods using the swallowing-without-chewing strategy as described. The Armonk Diet wants you to fill up on food without calories so that you can then eat whatever you like, in reasonable amounts, without desperate hunger cravings driving your need to binge eat. By the time you get to your second course, you should feel comfortable eating smaller portions.

Does this idea of swallowing food without first chewing it sound a little crazy to you? You are not alone. Altering your eating experience in such a fundamental way can seem strange at first. It certainly helps if you keep an open mind and a willingness to try new experiences. It helps even more to have the motivation of desperation due to previous failed attempts at losing weight.

Anyone can follow The Armonk Diet and succeed in losing weight. If I can do it, so can you. Just try it. Take the leap of faith. You may need time to adjust before you feel completely comfortable. Start as slowly as you need to. But try it, in the end. The Armonk Diet results in your hunger going away, with no net calories getting into your body, before you even begin eating what you want for the nutrition or pleasure phase of your meal. You have the power to decide how much you want to eat after you feel full, without hunger driving you to overeat or make poor food choices. You can decide in advance how much to eat, if you want, or just pick and choose from whatever is sitting around in your kitchen once you have filled up. Once your stomach is full, you have all the power to control your eating choices in a way that will lead to a thinner you, without hunger cravings driving poor eating choices.

We discussed earlier the ineffectiveness of exercise as a weight loss method. With The Armonk Diet, you have the opportunity for exercise to actually count toward your weight loss efforts. You will remember that the disadvantage of exercise is the increased appetite that exercise induces, which results in eating more, which negates the calorie burning from exercising. However, if you follow The Armonk Diet, you can swallow first course seeds as much as you need to, in order to satisfy your increased appetite for any reason, including after exercising. This results in no net weight gain, so the calories you burn during exercise can finally count toward your weight loss goal.

Chapter 9: Learning the Swallowing Technique

You now know that you can lose weight by swallowing unchewed seeds. Unchewed seeds will fill you up without affecting your weight, before you eat whatever you want afterwards. You have the ability to satisfy your appetite without worrying about the caloric consequences. Now comes the only obstacle to your success: learning the swallowing technique, which will determine whether your new eating method succeeds. Not everyone can swallow solid food without chewing it. If you can learn to swallow without chewing, you have an excellent chance to succeed at The Armonk Diet. But seed swallowing may present a challenge for some people and, for those who need the extra help, this chapter offers assistance in learning to swallow without chewing.

Coming to Terms with a New Swallowing Mindset

For most people, swallowing without chewing simply requires changing your mealtime thought process and getting used to a new routine. You can adapt to it pretty quickly with the proper motivation. Remember your goal of getting your weight under control and imagine the fabulous new you that will appear once you have achieved that goal.

Do you wonder if you will be able to swallow foods without first chewing them? Let's go back to basics and remember that you already swallow some things without chewing. For instance, you already swallow liquids without chewing them. But you also swallow some semisolid foods without chewing. You probably do not have to chew mostly-liquid and semi-solid foods such as soups, purees, oatmeal, custard, pudding, gelatin, and ice cream. All you will do in The Armonk Diet is slightly extend the range of what you can swallow without chewing. Whole kernel corn is soft enough, and wet enough, to practically be one of the semi-solid foods that you already swallow without giving it a second thought. And well-cooked beans are almost as soft, and would be a natural next step once you feel comfortable swallowing whole kernels of corn.

You will definitely need a little time to adjust to your new swallowing regimen. Swallowing intact seeds without first chewing them feels very different in your throat than swallowing chewed food. You will feel more of a scraping sensation in your throat than you normally experience when you swallow. Depending on your personal level of anxiety about swallowing, you may find it easy to plunge right in to your new regimen, or you may need to build up to it. Your success will depend on how well you swallow food in general, as well as on how well you handle the tactile sensation of seeds in your mouth and throat, specifically their hardness and roughness.

If the prospect of swallowing unchewed food makes you nervous, just remember that most of us swallow without much difficulty. Overweight individuals probably excel in the swallowing department, having become overweight in the first place by swallowing too much, too well. So swallowing a bunch of seeds might not present too great a challenge. Most people find corn and beans soft enough to swallow whole without much discomfort. If you do experience difficulty swallowing whole seeds, you can often overcome this hurdle with a little guidance and some practice. If you keep an open mind and persevere, you will probably succeed.

Mindfulness will play much more of a role in your new mealtime practices, at least in the beginning. Your old eating routine may not have required much conscious effort in order to put food in your mouth, chew it up, and swallow it. For those who eat on auto-pilot, your new routine will require paying attention to what you swallow, if only to remind yourself not to chew. After a while, it becomes automatic and you won't have to pay as much attention any more.

Teaching Yourself to Swallow Whole Seeds

Your next step is to try out the swallowing technique. To get started, if you consider yourself brave, just put a spoonful of whole kernel corn in your mouth and see if you can swallow it comfortably. If you succeeded, you don't need to bother with most of the rest of this chapter. If not, let's proceed further.

Can you easily swallow a pill? The answer can help predict how challenging you will find swallowing seeds. If you can swallow a pill easily, then you will probably not experience much difficulty swallowing seeds. However, up to a third of people cannot swallow pills well. Difficulty swallowing pills does not automatically mean you will fail at The Armonk Diet, since pills require more swallowing effort than seeds. So don't worry if you cannot swallow pills well. Canned whole kernel corn and well-cooked beans have a softer texture and a wetter exterior than pills, which makes them much easier to swallow than hard, dry pills. Most people, although not all, can swallow whole kernels of corn pretty easily.

If you can get to the point of comfortably swallowing a whole kernel of corn, you will probably eventually succeed at following The Armonk Diet. So your goal is to get to that point. If you do not feel comfortable swallowing a kernel of corn without first chewing it, you may benefit from some of the advice that follows. So let's get started.

Open a can of whole kernel corn and try to swallow a single kernel. Take your time. Did it go down easily and without discomfort? If yes, then you can skip to the last paragraph in this chapter. In fact, if you succeed at any step along the way, you can pretty much stop reading all the following swallowing suggestions and head straight to the last paragraph. Every next suggestion assumes you failed all the previous suggestions.

If you did not succeed, try heating up the corn kernels, which makes swallowing them a little less uncomfortable than serving them at room temperature. Try to swallow a heated corn kernel. Still unsuccessful? Don't give up.

Next, put another warm kernel of corn into your mouth, and let it rest on your tongue. Get used to the sensation. Roll it around in your mouth, but don't chew it. See if you can use

79

your tongue to work the corn toward the back of your mouth, and then try to swallow it. Did you find success? If it worked, skip to the last paragraph.

Still not successful? Try some lubrication to make the kernel more slippery inside your mouth. Get some olive oil, and try coating the kernel of corn with the olive oil. It won't stick to your tongue as much, and will slide down your throat more easily. If it worked, skip to the last paragraph.

No luck yet? Try wetting your mouth more. After you put a kernel of corn into your mouth, let it sit there for a little while, to give saliva a chance to accumulate in your mouth. Take a sip of water if you need to. Some people swallow pills this way. Swish the extra saliva or water around in your mouth to moisten the corn, which should make it easier to swallow. Try to swallow it again, mixed in with the saliva or water. If it worked, skip to the last paragraph.

Still not going down easily? Take a full gulp of water with the corn in your mouth, swish the water around in your mouth, try and get the kernel of corn to float in with the swishing water, and then try swallowing the water and corn together.

If you need to, add a corn kernel to some warm water in a soupspoon to make it more like soup, and try swallowing that. If you get to the point where you can swallow at least one kernel without chewing, then you have an accomplishment on which you can build, and you can skip to the last paragraph.

Still not successful? You can try either or both of the two tips below, adapted from suggestions for people who have trouble swallowing pills.

- Fill a non-rigid squeezable plastic water or soda bottle of any size with water. Put a kernel of corn in your mouth, and close your lips tightly around the opening of the bottle. Tilt your head slightly backwards and, keeping a seal between the bottle and your lips by pursing your lips, suck some water from the bottle. Swallow the water and the kernel of corn without letting air into the bottle as you swallow. You should see and hear the bottle collapse in on itself as you swallow.

- Put a kernel of corn on your tongue, and then take a medium sip of water, but do not swallow yet. Bend your head forward a little, swish the water around in your mouth, and let the corn kernel float around in it, and then swallow the kernel of corn and the water with your head bent forward.

If all of your corn swallowing attempts so far did not succeed, you could always try starting off swallowing something smaller than corn. This allows you to make progress so that you eventually build up to corn. Some people find it difficult to swallow whole objects like seeds because their throats reject the intrusion of the seeds and tense up. In order to overcome your throat's aversion to swallowing something the size of a kernel of corn, you can practice swallowing smaller objects to familiarize your throat with swallowing something whole.

You now have permission to try swallowing small candy instead. True, swallowing candy will not help you to lose weight. But focus on the mission at hand, trying to develop your swallowing skills. Since you can't follow The Armonk Diet without learning how to swallow, think of this as a necessary evil in the service of a greater good. Small candies that can help include sprinkles, mini M&Ms, and Nerds. Put a sprinkle in your mouth like a pill, and swallow it with a drink of water. If you cannot swallow a sprinkle on the first try, let it rest on your tongue and soften and melt a little. Then retry swallowing it. Repeat this until you feel comfortable with all the candies of this size. Next, try swallowing a slightly larger-sized candy such as a Skittle, regular M&M, jelly bean, or Tic Tac. Repeat the same procedure with this size until you feel comfortable. You should practice every day for about 10 minutes until you can swallow a piece of candy that's about the same size as a whole corn kernel. Once you achieve the ability to swallow a corn kernel-sized candy, you can go back to any of the previous paragraphs and try again with actual corn kernels.

If, after all that, you still can't swallow a kernel of corn without chewing it, perhaps you should consider scheduling a personal consultation with a swallowing therapist, or admit defeat and go to Plan B, discussed below. Ultimately, if you cannot swallow intact seeds smoothly and comfortably, you should not try to follow The Armonk Diet. Please do not try to force the seeds down your throat by swallowing unsafely. Forced swallowing raises your risk of aspiration, which is what happens when you choke down your food and it accidentally enters your windpipe (the breathing passage that leads into your lungs) instead of proceeding the usual way down your esophagus toward your stomach. Aspiration can lead to coughing, choking, and even death in rare cases. If you cannot swallow corn kernels comfortably despite trying to follow the recommendations above, feel free to keep trying the steps above until you succeed, but in the meantime please do not attempt this diet. Having said that, you might consider trying a less-effective variation of The Armonk Diet. Called Plan B, it allows you to eat in the usual way, including chewing everything before you swallow.

The Plan B Option

This second-best option, which allows chewing of all the food you consume, substitutes low-calorie plain vegetables for your first, seed-swallowing, course. For certain dieters, especially binge eaters who have a large amount of weight to drop, this will work almost as well as The Armonk Diet, without the precondition of having to swallow unchewed food. I added a table of nutrition information for common vegetables below, to show you that, for every vegetable on this list, you can eat virtually all you want without having much of an impact on your weight, because of the low calorie content of unprocessed vegetables. As an example, look at cauliflower, which has 25 calories in 3.5 ounces. That converts into about 115 calories per pound. So you could steam and eat 5 pounds of cauliflower as your substitute first course, which would add about 600 calories to your day's total. Granted, you would not have consumed those 600 calories while strictly following The Armonk Diet, but you will not find a lower total number of calories from just about any other food item. And if you choose your second course foods sensibly, your ultimate weight loss might come out the same. You don't have to choose cauliflower, if you don't like it. You can do the same calculation with any of the other vegetables on the list, and you will come up with a similar result. Whether you eat your chosen plain vegetables raw, steamed, or cooked until they turn to mush will make no difference to your weight loss outcome, and you will get the added bonus of the nutritional benefit of eating vegetables. If you select Plan B, you can skip the next few chapters and go straight to Chapter 13.

The Last Paragraph

Hopefully you reached this paragraph having determined that you can swallow at least one whole kernel of corn, even if you needed to lubricate that single kernel to get it to go down. If so, you now need to build on your success in order to work your way up to swallowing whole corn kernels by the spoonful. Gradually increase the number of corn kernels that you put in your mouth, starting with two at a time and proceeding from there, and practice swallowing progressively more until you can swallow an entire spoonful of corn kernels at once. Once can swallow a spoonful of corn kernels, you can feel confident about following The Armonk Diet. If you cannot swallow an entire spoonful, don't worry. When you have mastered the technique of swallowing a few kernels at a time, it just gets easier with more practice. You may need to eat more slowly than usual in the beginning as you focus on how you swallow. This could work in your favor, because slower meal consumption leads you to fill up on less food. As you improve your ability to swallow without chewing, you will start filling yourself up and losing weight. Once you start seeing results, the positive feedback will increase your motivation to further improve your swallowing technique. Now get ready to lose some weight!

Vegetables Serving Size (gram weight/ounce weight)	Calories
Asparagus 5 spears (93 g/3.3 oz)	20
Bell Pepper 1 medium (148 g/5.3 oz)	25
Broccoli 1 medium stalk (148 g/5.3 oz)	45
Carrot 1 carrot, 7" long, 1 1/4" diameter (78 g/2.8 oz)	30
Cauliflower 1/6 medium head (99 g/3.5 oz)	25
Celery 2 medium stalks (110 g/3.9 oz)	15
Cucumber 1/3 medium (99 g/3.5 oz)	10
Green (Snap) Beans 3/4 cup cut (83 g/3.0 oz)	20
Green Cabbage 1/12 medium head (84 g/3.0 oz)	25

Table. Calorie Content of Vegetables

Chapter 10: Beans

Whole kernel corn's size and consistency make it the most comfortable choice for swallowing. If you want to keep your dieting program simple and easy, you can't beat whole kernel corn as your designated first-course seed of choice. However, the same-old same-old routine of filling yourself up with all-corn all the time might eventually make you ponder other options. If first-course boredom does not bother you, just stick with whole kernel corn. You will have a simpler life that way, since buying corn requires very little effort beyond carrying freezer bags or cans home from the market and storing them somewhere. But if you despise swallowing corn all the time, just want to diversify your dieting technique, or cherish a little more variety in your diet, beans can make things ever-so-slightly more interesting.

You can achieve the same results and follow the same diet technique with swallowing beans either in addition to, or instead of, corn. Although beans have a different consistency than corn, you can still swallow them easily, just not quite as easily as corn. If you prepare and swallow beans following the techniques in this book, your body will not digest them. If you have a special reason why you cannot swallow corn, such as food sensitivities or difficulty finding a corn supplier, feel free to follow The Armonk Diet using beans. Otherwise, you should try corn first, and wait until you have gotten used to corn, and have successfully lost some weight, before tackling beans.

Beans give you more choices during your first course, but not necessarily more flavor. You might think that different types of beans would have different flavors, but not really. A taste test of all the different dried beans in the market determined that all beans taste pretty much the same if you prepare them the same way. They taste like nothing, at least when you swallow them whole. With whole kernel corn, you can taste an element of sweetness (if you buy the unsalted version) or saltiness. Although beans lack any interesting flavor, they do have the same weight-losing effectiveness as corn. For the flavor mavens among you, don't despair, you can flavor them if you desire, by following the suggestions in Chapter 12. But you don't need to bother going to great lengths to improve your first-course taste experience, since your primary goal is satiety during your first course rather than food enjoyment. Your dining pleasure comes during your second course. Since the variety of bean makes no real difference in terms of flavor or weight loss results, feel free to buy the cheapest beans sold at your regular market or warehouse store, and stock up.

For your first bean experience, you should try frozen soybeans. You can purchase frozen soybeans (also known by the Japanese name edamame) shelled and unsalted, and you don't need to soak or cook them. Just microwave them until warm, for up to a few minutes if you start with an entire package straight from the freezer, after which you can swallow them whole. Check their firmness after you heat them. If too mushy, they will break apart when you swallow them, which will lead to digestion and failure to lose weight. If your throat feels uncomfortable due to dryness when you swallow heated frozen soybeans, add some water or vegetable oil (I recommend olive oil) to the container to lubricate them. The potential downsides of swallowing soybeans include their relatively high cost compared to other types of beans and the need to store them in your freezer.

Canned whole beans constitute a reasonable option. The manufacturer saved you all the work of soaking and cooking these beans. The convenience of opening a can and the ease of swallowing whole cooked beans appear at first glance to make them a great choice, as long as you don't mind their saltiness. Most canned beans contain ridiculous amounts of salt (unsalted brands cost more and can prove hard to find).

The other disadvantage of canned beans relates to their seed coats' integrity. Canned cooked beans often split apart due to their mushiness, and some canned beans have broken seed coats. Around 15% of beans in a typical can will be broken, exposing their interiors to your digestive processes and ultimately to calorie absorption, not to mention the stereotypical gassiness that often follows eating beans. You might recognize that digestion occurred, after the fact, when you start passing more gas than usual. Undigested beans, on the other hand, do not cause excessive gassiness. As a remedy, if you purchase canned beans, you could take the time to inspect them and pick out and discard the broken ones, but then you lose much of the advantage of saving on preparation time.

Certain beans that stay relatively intact in their cans include red kidney beans, pigeon peas and sometimes lima beans. You have to inspect them and make a judgement. For the goal of weight loss, and for reduced farting, their seed coats should remain intact.

Preparing Your Own Beans

At some point, you may decide you want to prepare your own beans. Perhaps you dislike the expense involved in buying freezer packages of soybeans or crave more control over the saltiness and fragility of canned beans, and wonder if you can do a better job yourself. Yes, you can. Preparing your own beans will save you money in the long run, and will give you absolute control over how your beans look and taste, but will require extra work on your part. A little bit of obsessiveness helps.

You can start with dried beans purchased from your local supermarket or warehouse store. The typical supermarket sells beans in one pound bags, usually for less than $2. One local warehouse store sells ten-pound bags of beans for $6-10, and another big-box retailer has 4-pound bags for about $3. Unfortunately, they are not always available, so you might want to stock up once you realize this method works for you.

Now comes the work. The beans need to soak, and you may want to cook them, depending on your preference, which we will discuss in upcoming pages. Then you have to rinse them off, transfer them into containers and store them. If you do all this, you won't have to deal with the various disadvantages of pre-cooked beans outlined above, and you may also find it strangely satisfying to prepare your beans yourself. If you do undertake bean self-preparation, you will want to make the largest batch practical each time, in order to maximize your time efficiency. Storage of each batch will probably generate complaints from anyone who needs to share your refrigerator or freezer, since your beans will take up a lot of space. The rest of this chapter details the steps of preparing your own beans.

You can choose to prepare your beans to a preferred consistency, either relatively soft or hard. Either way, you want them as intact as possible to prevent digestion. Soft beans enable easier swallowing, but require longer cooking. Unfortunately, longer cooking tends to break the seed coat, which makes cooked beans more digestible, which you don't want. If you have special bean-cooking skills and know how to cook beans without disrupting their seed coats, you absolutely should cook them. If you consider yourself an average bean cooker without bean-whispering capabilities and wish to reduce your beans' digestibility, you should cook them less than usual, or not at all. Less cooking means less digestibility and fewer broken beans. So ideally, you would not cook them at all, which saves you a lot of time and effort, and results in the beans having a harder, very firm texture. Uncooked beans may therefore feel more uncomfortable than their cooked counterparts in your throat when swallowed. Whether you cook your beans or not, you still have to soak them, though. Cooked, undercooked, or uncooked? They can all work for you. It's good to have choices!

You might want to consider soaked, uncooked beans as a less time-consuming, and more practical, alternative to cooking your beans for purposes of The Armonk Diet. However, there is no scientific literature to either support or warn against swallowing uncooked beans in this way so, if you do it, it's at your own risk. Fortunately, uncooked (but well-soaked and thoroughly rinsed) beans appear safe for human consumption based on my personal experience. Despite their hardness, uncooked beans' smoothness makes them easy to swallow with some lubrication from water or a little bit of olive oil. As an unexpected extra bonus, even with broken seed coats, uncooked beans, swallowed unchewed, do not seem to undergo digestion or cause the gassiness usually associated with eating cooked beans.

There are two potential food-safety exceptions to the option of swallowing soaked, uncooked, beans: kidney beans and their relatives, cannellini beans. Both types of beans could potentially cause food poisoning if *eaten* undercooked, due to a plant toxin that both beans contain, which requires cooking to inactivate. So in the case of kidney beans and cannellini beans, you should cook them. We will discuss this issue more a little later.

Apart from the kidney/cannellini bean toxicity issue, you may also wish to cook your beans because you desire the softer consistency that cooking gives them, or because you have concerns about the possibility of ill health that could result from eating raw foods in general. Theoretically, germs such as bacteria, mold, and parasites can coat the surfaces of raw foods. Germophobes may prefer the safer option of cooking their beans, or just stick to using frozen soybeans and canned beans. Just remember the downsides of cooked beans, including extra preparation time; and broken seed coats, which can lead to digestion, causing flatulence and unnecessary weight gain.

Now let's spend some time discussing do-it-yourself bean preparation. You will save money, if not time, and you will retain the greatest control over the flavor, texture, and intactness of your beans. Bean preparation usually involves three steps: soaking, rinsing, and cooking. Raw (uncooked) beans only require soaking and rinsing, and don't necessarily need a stove. Undercooked and fully cooked beans require a heat source such as a stove or hotplate. Undercooking your beans offers a middle ground between soaked-only and fully cooked beans, making undercooked beans a little softer than soaked-only beans and therefore easier to swallow; resulting in less cracked seed coats than fully cooked beans; killing more of the germs on the beans' surface than with soaked-only beans; and, in the case of kidney or cannellini beans, inactivating the toxin mentioned above that could potentially cause food poisoning.

Soaking

All dry beans need soaking. For the easiest bean-soaking method, use the Overnight Cold Soak. You let your chosen beans soak in a pot filled with water for at least several hours, typically overnight. You should first pick out any broken beans and stones that you notice in the package. Make the ratio of water to beans in the pot at least 3:1, because the beans will absorb a lot of the water. Beans enlarge to two to three times their dry size after soaking. A half-pound of beans will almost fill up a quart container, once you soak it well. In a 12 quart pot, you can add up to 6 pounds of beans, and then fill up the rest of the pot with water, almost to the top. Filling the pot with hot water from the faucet seems to work a little more quickly than using straight cold water, if you want a slightly faster turnaround time before you proceed to the next step.

For the fastest, albeit more labor-intensive, option try a Quick Hot Soak. Add the same amount of water to a pot, then add the beans, and bring the water to a boil for at least 2 minutes, then let stand until cool, usually a few hours at most. You can save a few minutes of heating time by filling the pot with hot water from your faucet, rather than cold.

Preparing Soaked, Uncooked Beans

This method saves time, since you do not have to cook anything, but requires extra labor during the rinsing off process, in order to rid the soaked beans of as much field residue as possible. With both the cold or hot soak methods, once the beans have plumped up enough, you need to rinse them off. You should not just run a little tap water over them and pronounce the job done. Instead, drain off the soak water by pouring all your beans into a colander, rinse the remaining dirt and residue from the soaking pot, return the drained beans back into the soaking pot (or a new clean container to reduce contamination), and refill the bean-filled container with tap water. Shake or stir the container for a minute or so, then drain the beans off again, and rinse out the container again. Repeat this up to several times until no foam or froth appears in the water after you shake or stir the container, and until the water appears clear. The foam, froth, and general muddiness of the rinse water indicate the presence of field residue from the bean picking process, including germs, dirt and fertilizer. Warm or hot water seems to outperform cold water in rinsing-off effectiveness. Hand stir instead of spoon stirring if you want to keep as many seed coats intact as possible, but remember that intact seed coats may prove unimportant in the case of uncooked beans.

You may find shaking more efficient than stirring. Using a sealable container that you can shake will take less overall time than hand-stirring, but you need to have the ability to lift a heavy container and shake it around. Each time you repeat the cycle of draining the beans into a colander, then rinsing the soaking container, then pouring the beans back into the container, then re-adding water, then hand-stirring or shaking the container for a minute or two, the water in the container should turn less turbid and foamy, indicating your success in rinsing off ever-greater amounts of field residue. At some point, usually after three or so cycles of rinsing, or whenever you decide to quit due to muscle fatigue or boredom, the rinse water will appear clear enough. Now you can drain the beans one last time, and then go on to the next step of portioning them out into smaller, single-serving containers that you can seal and put in your refrigerator or freezer for storage until you are ready to use them. Between rinsing the beans and the subsequent clean-up, this time consuming process still takes less time than cooking. It takes me about 30 minutes to rinse off, portion out, and do the cleanup for, ten pounds of soaked dry beans. The other difference between soaking-only and cooking is that cooking kills all the potential germs in the field residue, so does not require the several cycles of rinsing with manual pot-stirring and container-shaking.

If you plan on storing your soaked beans for longer than several days in a refrigerator, consider the possibility that they might eventually spoil. Check your beans for a sour smell, mucus-like coating, sprouting, and bubbles, and discard them if they seem spoiled. On the other hand, you can expect frozen beans to keep almost indefinitely. So if you have the freezer room and enough containers, keep a few days' supply in your refrigerator, and the rest in the freezer.

If you want a sealable container to shake your beans during the rinsing off procedure, you can find a relatively large, partly water-tight container called a 16.91 qt. Smart Locks Keep Box Crystal Clear at The Container Store for under $20. It does not actually stay water-tight once you start shaking it vigorously, so I recommend shaking it in or over your sink, and not turning it upside down while you shake it. If you hold the lid on tightly with your hands while shaking it, the seal will hold water inside much more effectively. As a side note, between one of these containers and a 12-quart soup pot, you should be able to fully soak at least 14 pounds of dried beans, putting about eight pounds in the Keep Box, and another 6 in the 12-quart pot. One ten-pound bag of dry beans will ultimately yield about 17 quarts of soaked beans.

If you have white walls and counters, and favor dark-colored beans such as black beans, you might want to know that some of their color comes off in the soak water and rinse water. This knowledge may come in handy when you plan to pour off the soak and rinse water into a colander in your sink and then notice that the splatter from the water has stained your nearby walls and countertops the color of your beans. In order to save yourself extra time and effort cleaning up, consider taking special care when you rinse dark beans, or using a bean whose color you wouldn't mind seeing splattered on your walls and counters.

Cooking Your Beans

Cooking your beans makes them softer, which makes them more easily swallowable than soaked-only beans. It takes longer than soaking-only, but you avoid some of the manual labor involved in rinsing off the beans several times to wash off the field residue. In addition, if you have a suppressed immune system for any reason, you should cook your beans just to avoid the possibility that any germs present in the field contamination might cause an infection that your body can't fight off. When you decide to cook your beans, you can start by pouring off the soak water and beans into a colander, and just lightly rinse the beans before they go into a cooking pot. You can cook them in the pot you soaked them in, if you rinse it out first.

Add the beans to your cooking pot, and pour water over them so the liquid covers them by at least 2 inches. Bring the water to a boil, and then turn down the heat. Simmer your soaked beans on low to medium heat so you barely see any bubbling, usually for between 45 minutes and 2 hours. The more gently they simmer, the less broken they will be at the end. Skim any foam from the top of the pot periodically, mostly for the first several minutes until your beans boil, but also at the end. Stir the beans periodically while they cook so that they don't stick to the bottom of your pot. Cooking times will vary depending on which variety of bean you cook. Typical guidelines:

Black beans	1 hour
Great northern beans	45 - 60 minutes
Light/dark red kidney beans	1 ½ - 2 hours
Navy beans	1 ½ - 2 hours
Pinto beans	1 ½ - 2 hours

You can test the doneness of your beans by mashing them with a fork or between your fingers. You want your beans tender but not mushy. If your beans remain crunchy or underdone after simmering for the recommended cooking time, continue cooking them, checking their consistency every 10-15 minutes until done.

Once done, let your beans cool off and then package them in single-serving containers to store in your refrigerator or freezer. The mushier the beans, the more they will break apart during the transfer process. Cooked beans, if refrigerated, will keep for up to five days in a tightly covered storage container. Frozen, they should keep almost forever. Do not store your cooked beans in their cooking pot.

Cleaning up after cooking your beans may prove dirtier and more time consuming than just soaking them, but at least you won't have to spend as much time manually stirring the soaked beans or shaking their rinse container.

Undercooked Beans

Undercooked beans occupy a middle ground between uncooked and fully cooked beans. If you follow the above instructions but stop boiling after, say, 30 minutes, you will cook your beans enough to kill germs and inactivate toxins. These undercooked beans will also be a little softer than if uncooked, but more intact than when fully cooked. This might prove a good choice for those who want a compromise between the benefits of cooked and uncooked beans, such as fans of kidney or cannellini beans who prefer their beans on the uncooked side but who also want to not worry about food safety.

Kidney and Cannellini Beans

Kidney beans and their close relatives, cannellini beans, require special preparation, in theory. You can eat these two bean varieties safely if you cook them, but they could potentially give you food poisoning if you eat them without fully cooking them. They contain phytohemagglutinin, a toxic substance that can cause severe abdominal pain, vomiting, and diarrhea, and which you can only inactivate by cooking. This warning applies to *eating* raw or undercooked kidney beans and cannellini beans. No one has ever researched the specific question of swallowing them without chewing, so they might be safe, but swallow them uncooked only at your own risk. I personally experienced no food-poisoning problems by following the soak-only preparation method with kidney beans. But since no data yet exists regarding the safety of swallowing whole uncooked kidney and cannellini beans, you should avoid consuming them in any not-fully-cooked form out of an abundance of caution. With so many other bean options, why take a chance? If you want do-it-yourself uncooked beans, you can easily bypass kidney and cannellini beans, and none of the other bean types cause toxicity.

If you really want to incorporate kidney and cannellini beans into The Armonk Diet, just cook them, at least for long enough to inactive the toxin. As long as you do not mind the extra preparation time and labor, soak and then rinse them as described for all the other beans. Then, bring them to a boil in fresh water, on maximum heat. Once the water boils, turn the heat down to a gentle boil, which helps preserve the beans' seed coats. Let the beans boil gently for at least 30 minutes before you turn off the heat. Thirty minutes of boiling should be more than enough time to detoxify the phytohemagglutinin. Then you can transfer the beans gently into containers for storage. As a result of the long cooking time, some of your beans will probably fragment, meaning you will probably digest some of them. Don't use slow cookers (the kinds of pots that cook food at low temperatures for several hours) to cook these beans because slow cookers don't get hot enough to destroy the toxin. Ultimately, due to the toxicity issue, neither kidney nor cannellini beans make great choices for The Armonk Diet unless you fully cook them.

Reheating Your Beans

You can reheat your beans in a microwave if desired. Use whatever power setting and time you find will heat up the beans sufficiently without making them explode. As an example, using a one-quart container coming straight out of a refrigerator, 3-4 minutes on high should heat the beans pretty well. After heating the beans, you should rinse them again until you see no foam in the rinse water. Typically, the soaked-only beans will still have some foam to rinse off, in contrast to the less-foamy cooked beans.

You can successfully prepare many types of dried beans, such as those usually stocked at your local market, using this method. Some examples include baby lima beans, Central American red beans, Roman beans, whole green peas, small red beans, black beans, and pinto beans. You can soak black eyed peas, but I would not cook them because their seed coats come off too easily.

Storage of Dry Beans

You can keep dry beans for up to a year in an airtight container in a cool, dry environment, away from direct sunlight. This helps them to avoid turning rancid or changing their consistency. During storage, beans may either absorb or lose moisture, which can affect their soaking and cooking time, but this does not matter much if their destiny is to be swallowed whole. If stored longer than 12 months, or exposed to unfavorable storage conditions, beans may never soften sufficiently, no matter how long they soak or cook. On the other hand, some beans can cook up tender after years of storage.

Bean Quirks and Tips

You will find undercooked and raw soaked beans harder to swallow than their cooked counterparts. Even if you usually swallow an entire soup-spoon full of whole kernel corn at once, you might reasonably expect to comfortably swallow only a few or several beans at a time, depending on their size. Swallowing too many uncooked beans at once will scrape your throat. Adding two teaspoons of olive oil to a one- or two-quart container of beans makes swallowing them much more pleasant. If you do not want to oil your beans, you can soften them a different way. Just mix in a portion of whole kernel corn. With enough corn mixed in, the overall softness of what goes into your mouth improves, and the beans become much easier to swallow. Another remedy for uncomfortable bean swallowing, taking a large sip of water after you put the beans in your mouth, will also help you swallow them more quickly and easily.

As you get more comfortable swallowing ever-larger spoonfuls of beans during your first course, you might also notice that, occasionally, a small piece of what you swallow gets stuck in your throat. You will swallow most of the spoonful, but a little piece of a broken bean or a seed coat that separated from its underlying bean will catch and stick in your throat momentarily, and you may need to clear your throat to spit it out. Seed coats can separate from their seeds during soaking, cooking or swallowing, and the seed coat by itself often just curls up and does not pass smoothly down your throat. Do not let this scare you. Just take a sip of water and try to swallow it back down, or spit it out.

Seed Varieties to Avoid

You should avoid some other seed types, listed below, that do not work well for various reasons.

Lentils

Lentils can frustrate you. You will struggle to swallow hard lentils, so you have to soak them for a while. However, if you wait until they soften too much, they plump up and burst right through their seed coats, and you will digest them completely. Somewhere, a middle ground exists, and it's a fine line. After soaking for most of the day in cold water, they soften a little bit, but they still feel unpleasantly rough in your mouth when you swallow them. As a result, you will probably want to lubricate them, perhaps with something soupy, or to coat them with some olive oil or a sauce. They also tend to get stuck in your throat, which may lead you to aspirate them and choke. You have better things to do than to waste your time trying to make lentils fit into this regimen.

Dried Barley

Dried barley, a cereal grain, looks like a seed in its package, and sits next to all the other beans in the supermarket, but does not work with The Armonk Diet. Don't let it fool you. You will digest dried barley.

Dried Split Peas

Dried split peas have no seed coat and only work if you do not cook them to the point of softness. Once softened, you digest them just like regular food. You could perform a Quick Hot Soak, with 2 minutes of boiling, but you would have to cool down the split peas after only 15 minutes of hot soaking. Split peas that you prepare in this manner will remain pretty hard, which means that your throat will probably feel uncomfortable if you try swallowing them unlubricated. You will probably discover that you can only swallow a few at a time without taking a sip of water to help them go down. With a little water in your mouth, you can swallow the hard split peas easily. But with the other bean types, and with corn, you generally won't need to take the extra sip of water. So don't bother with split peas, because they require extra work, which takes away from the "ridiculously easy" spirit of The Armonk Diet. You can make this method work, but who needs the aggravation?

Chapter 11: How to Do The Armonk Diet

Now that you know the theory behind The Armonk Diet, it's time to put it into action. To recap, you can only lose weight if you reduce your calorie intake to less than what your body needs to maintain itself. Dieting, alone among all the potential do-it-yourself weight reduction options, offers your best chance to successfully slim down. The Armonk Diet offers you the easiest and most effective way to diet, without leaving you hungry or depriving you of foods you love. You will spoil your appetite by filling yourself up at the start of every meal or snack with real food that you can buy cheaply at just about any market and, if you swallow it without chewing, the calories won't count. Since you won't have much room left in your stomach after you spoil your appetite, your drive to keep eating will diminish. When you have filled up sufficiently, no longer driven by hunger cravings, you can eat whatever other food you want for pleasure or nutrition purposes.

You can choose to lose weight quickly or slowly by varying the ratio of the amounts of food in each course. You will determine your optimal weight loss velocity through a trial and error process. Slow weight loss offers you the best chance to maintain your health and successfully maintain your weight in the long term. As you ease into The Armonk Diet, your first courses will probably start with just a small amount of whole kernel corn per meal as you try out the technique before you fully commit to it. Then you will gradually increase the amount of corn you swallow, while gradually decreasing the amount of food you eat in your second course. For rapid weight loss, you will maximize your first-course indigestible seed consumption and minimize or eliminate your second-course digestible food consumption. If you want to attempt maximum rapid weight loss, please pay special attention to the warning about starvation fasting in Chapter 4, as well as to the nutrition recommendations in Chapter 15, in order to maintain your health. Rapid weight reduction will not serve you well in the long run.

Getting Started

Your first course, during which you will mostly or completely fill yourself up, consists of seeds that you swallow without chewing. Aside from the novelty of swallowing your food unchewed, you will find the logistics of eating pretty simple. Your initial seed of choice, whole kernel corn, far surpasses other types of seeds in both ease of swallowing and availability, and makes following The Armonk Diet a breeze.

You can use canned whole kernel corn, or you can buy the bagged whole kernel corn in your supermarket's freezer section.

Most dieters will obtain their best results by filling themselves up as much as possible at the start of all meals and snacks. Do not feel compelled to eat a second course when you have satisfied your hunger after filling yourself up enough after your first course. You can designate some of your meals and snacks as first-course-only affairs, although you should plan at least one second course every day in order to meet your body's nutrition requirements. When you select what to eat during your second course for nutrition or pleasure purposes, you should choose your calories carefully, although you can eat whatever you like. You can include junk food and high calorie-density items in your second courses with The Armonk Diet if you just can't help yourself, but you will lose more weight with healthier foods, not to mention avoiding the health risks of eating junk foods. If you seriously want to lose weight, you should eat for good health, too.

Although no absolute restrictions exist regarding what you can eat during your second course, you should minimize or avoid foods which contribute to hunger and cravings. These foods include comfort foods such as anything with added sugar; starchy foods such as bakery goods, cereals, rice, noodles, pizza, potatoes, and bread; salty prepared foods, because salt increases your appetite and encourages you to increase your food consumption; and calorie-dense items, such as nuts and chocolate, simply because they do not promote losing weight. The Armonk Diet can work even if you consume such appetite-provoking foods, but you will achieve better results if you skip them. But just to be clear, you can eat any and all of these things, if you must. Just make sure that, by the time you eat a second course that contains these less-than-desirable foods, you feel so full from your first course that you have lost your desire to eat any more. Make sure your hunger has significantly diminished before you begin your second course, so if you do succumb to the temptation to eat less-than-healthy foods, you can limit them to small quantities. Since you should already feel full after your first course, you should not have to gorge yourself on bad-for-you comfort and junk foods. Smarter yet, don't keep these foods at home in the first place. Choose fresh fruit as your healthiest option for dessert, if you need to end your meal on a sweet note.

Some second-course choices that offer a better chance at satiety than others include foods with high levels of protein, dietary fiber and water. Protein-rich foods (fish, meat, baked beans, lentils and eggs) and carbohydrate-rich foods (pasta, rice, wholegrain breads and cereals) satisfy the most. Fruit and vegetables, especially boiled potatoes, have high satiety values, whereas bakery products such as biscuits, cakes, and croissants satisfy the least. While protein seems to stave off hunger for longer than carbohydrates, fat exerts the weakest effects on satiety. This probably explains why high fat diets often lead to over-eating, which results in weight gain.

If you can, try to plan in advance what and how much food you want to eat during your second course, regardless of who prepares your food. Studies show that, in food-ordering situations, pre-planners subconsciously consider how their meal will affect their health, and tend to choose lower-calorie meals. In contrast, those who order food just before they eat primarily think about how good the food will taste, and less about the health impact of their choices, so they order less-healthy items. Advance meal planning takes a little more discipline, but lets you avoid the poor food choices made by hungry eaters driven by their cravings. Just as you can make poor food choices under the stress of severe hunger, so can you lose control of your best weight-control impulses when you make spur-of-the-moment eating decisions during a meal.

Remember, you want to feel full, or very close to full, following your first course, so your second course revolves mostly around the specific goals of nutrition and pleasure, not quantity. You can enjoy decadent food by eating very small amounts of it, once you feel full enough from your first course.

During your second course, you shouldn't stuff yourself past the point of fullness. If you regularly find yourself overeating despite feeling completely full, and assuming you don't already have your own way of correcting this, you can address it in a few different ways. First, increase your first course quantities, so the overeating won't affect your weight as much. Second, pre-plan smaller second courses, and only eat what you set out for yourself in advance, and then stop. Third, go back to first course foods if you feel compelled to keep eating even after you have eaten enough second course foods. Don't feel obligated to clean your plate if you don't feel the need to eat any more. Since you control how much to eat during your second course, if you happen to set aside too much food, and recognize that you no longer need to eat, just stop, and put all the extra food away, saving it for a later meal.

If you prefer not to feel overstuffed and ready to burst after your meals, you have some other options for ways to stop eating before you fill up excessively. You could, for instance, incorporate slow eating, and put down your eating utensil for a few seconds between bites. That way, you have to consciously decide that you want the next bite of food, which can help break the cycle of shoveling food in your mouth without thinking about it. Chew your food thoroughly until it's not there anymore. Drink water during your meal, taking sips between each spoonful or bite; water quenches thirst better than flavored drinks. Drinking water, chewing thoroughly, and putting down your utensil between bites all force you to slightly delay your food consumption, leading to earlier satiety with less food consumption and less risk of feeling overstuffed.

You should start to feel your hunger diminish during your first course. Then pay attention to how long after that it takes for you to begin to feel satisfied. Then notice how much more time it takes before you feel full, and then how much more until you feel stuffed. Those times often remain relatively consistent from one day to the next. You can use them to know when the time has come to take an eating break to see if your hunger has finally been satisfied. Once the cravings disappear, your need to continue eating should also dissipate.

If you really like to feast and don't get full quickly, your main meal of the day might last two hours. As long as you do not take breaks during the meal, you don't have to rush or worry about taking too long. If you rest after your first course, you will lose your feeling of fullness before you start eating your second course, which will result in you eating more than you should. Assuming you plan to eat a second course, you should start as soon as you finish your first course. Just try not to take so much time eating your whole meal that your stomach starts to empty. An emptying stomach might make you lose your feeling of fullness and get a second wind, which you may misinterpret as a signal to continue eating second-course foods. So if you experience the return of your appetite during a prolonged meal, you probably need to start over and go back to first-course foods.

If you tend to follow a regular dining routine, for instance by eating at home every night, you will eventually realize roughly how much total food you need to consume during both courses. Try not to reach "completely full." Try to go for "enough." If you can reach "enough," then within a few minutes of stopping you will probably recognize that you actually feel pretty stuffed. Do not feel compelled to consume any particular quantity of food during either course. Just make sure you follow the nutritional guidelines regarding adequate daily nutrient consumption during your second course, which we will discuss in Chapter 15.

Sometimes, you can eat a whole meal, both courses, have a full belly, and still feel like you need to keep eating. Intellectually, you *know* you have eaten enough, but you still feel like you need a little something more. The bliss of meal satisfaction has not set in yet, despite eating a meal that has lasted for, in some cases, well over an hour. For those who need to lose weight, this frequent problem occurs because of the delay getting your brain to register eating satisfaction, even when your stomach feels near-ready to burst. This end-of-meal dilemma can lead to unnecessary extra food consumption. In the worst case scenario, you continue eating when you really don't need to, leading you to feel uncomfortably over-stuffed. You can deal with this situation in one of two ways: delay, or keep eating.

The delay option means you push away from the table and try walking around or sitting in a different location for just a few minutes. Sometimes you just need a brief break from sitting in front of food, and that brief delay will give your brain time to process the fact that you have finally lost your desire to eat.

This option is preferable to the keep-eating option, and will save your stomach some unnecessary pain.

If you choose to keep eating, you should consider returning to your first-course eating strategy. You could open up another can of whole kernel corn, and just swallow it as you did during your first course. Although the thought of going back to first-course techniques will probably not seem appealing, it would work if you did it. Swallow all the whole corn kernels you want until you finally lose your desire to eat.

As a second choice for further grazing, you might choose to eat healthy, low-calorie options such as raw vegetables. Baby carrots can fill that role nicely. You can buy baby carrots prewashed in a bag and just open them up and start nibbling them without any preparation, almost as conveniently as eating snack chips and pretzels. If the thought of eating raw carrots does not appeal to you, consider that you may not really need more food.

You might also consider snacking on an air-popped bowl of popcorn. Why popcorn? Popcorn, a so-called high satiety food, helps you feel fuller than many other foods without much caloric cost. And seeing a big bowl of popcorn mentally tricks you into thinking you get to eat a large portion. Also, it takes a while to eat a large bowl of popcorn, which gives your brain even more time to lose your desire to eat.

If you don't enjoy raw vegetables or popcorn, but want something else to munch on at the end of a non-quite finished meal, consider plain cereal grains. Raw or cooked oats, puffed rice, puffed wheat, puffed corn, and puffed millet can all be eaten with low calorie intake. Flavored cereals, on the other hand, typically have lots of added sugar, which contributes extra calories that you don't need. Non-sugared and unsalted popular cereals such as shredded wheat can fit in well, too, but their extra fiber, on top of an eating regimen that already causes frequent bowel movements, might make you run to the bathroom too frequently for comfort.

Still need to eat more? Repeat the following directions. Drink some water. Sit and wait a few minutes. Walk around. Swallow more whole kernel corn. Have another bowl of air-popped popcorn or plain cereal. Scarf down some more carrots. At some point, you will reach satiety nirvana, and lose the desire to eat any more, so you can comfortably stop.

You should avoid eating where you can see an electronic screen, especially a television, smartphone or computer screen. Focusing on a screen while eating will distract you and prolong your meal, thus preventing you from recognizing satiety. Even reading a book or newspaper while you eat can cause a similar distraction.

Your weight loss may plateau at some point. You may have reached your new set point, your body's limit on what you can accomplish using The Armonk Diet. But you may also just need to adjust the ratios of food consumed in your first and second courses. You can always try increasing the amount of indigestible first course food, and reduce the second course quantity in order to jump start further weight loss.

Now you know the essentials of The Armonk Diet. Perhaps it still sounds a little unnatural or just plain insane, this idea of not chewing foods before swallowing them. Reasonable people may hesitate to follow this method, which differs greatly from nature's usual way of eating. But take it from a believer, you can make this simple change if you want to. You will find this method easiest if you eat alone. However, if you eat with others, your dining companions will get used to your new routine soon, although they may kid you about it. Think of your motivation, all the reasons why you want to lose weight, and imagine how much better you will look and feel when you finally shed the pounds you want to lose. Perhaps you tried other methods of losing weight, and they did not work. Perhaps you had long ago given up, and never thought you would find a healthy way to lose weight. You didn't want to take dangerous medications or supplements, undergo surgery, or endure food restrictions that would make your life miserable. This method can work for you, if you try it. You may even start to see results within the first week, although it could take longer and, as they say, your results may vary.

The very first time you try to swallow seeds without chewing may make you nervous. You may wonder about the safety of eating this way. If you experience any anxiety, then make your debut as easy as possible by starting slowly with small amounts of corn kernels and lubricating them with plenty of water, which will make the swallowing experience similar to eating soup, or try the other suggestions from Chapter 9, where we discussed the swallowing technique. Later, as your swallowing confidence increases, you can drain the liquid off before swallowing.

You should now try The Armonk Diet on your own.

What to Expect

You might guess that, now that you have a good idea as to how to proceed with your new diet, nothing unexpected will happen. Well, not exactly. You should definitely expect a learning curve, so let's talk a little about various minor occurrences that may happen as you get started with The

Armonk Diet. There are a few aspects of following The Armonk Diet that you might want to know in advance. Specifically, how your nose and throat will feel, and what changes you may notice regarding your bowel habits.

Nasal Regurgitation

Let's take a moment for a brief anatomy recap so we can discuss nasal regurgitation. When you swallow, food passes from your mouth down your throat, then into your esophagus, until it eventually reaches your stomach. Notice that your nose did not participate in that discussion. But did you know that the back of your nose connects with your throat? If you don't believe me, look back at the Figure at the start of Chapter 3, and look for the nasal cavity. Your nose and throat passages connect in the back of your mouth.

Did you ever suddenly start laughing in the middle of swallowing something? If so, you may recall the feeling of the food or liquid you were trying to swallow going up and tickling the back of your nose. After you finally controlled your laughter, typically the food went back down into your throat, but it might also have come out your nose. That's called nasal regurgitation, and it can happen sometimes when you do not pay enough attention to swallowing. Although nasal regurgitation is unlikely if you concentrate on swallowing, once you get comfortable with your new swallowing method and lapse into your usual automatic food-shoveling mode, you may find yourself occasionally swallowing too many seeds at once. This may lead to episodes of nasal regurgitation as some of the seeds you try to swallow go up into the back of your nose instead of directly down your throat. This typically just tickles the back of your nose. Most of the time, whatever goes up into the back of your nose just falls naturally back down your throat, and you swallow it. Sometimes, however, you might sneeze out a kernel of corn, or you might blow your nose and see a corn kernel or bean come out. This harmless phenomenon serves as a reminder for you to pay more attention to swallowing or to reduce the quantity of seeds you try to swallow at once.

Nasal regurgitation will probably happen to you eventually, so don't let it get you upset the first time you experience it. The mucus in your nose will not poison your food, alter the taste of it, or spoil it, and you can swallow without worry any food that regurgitates up into your nose. You can avoid nasal regurgitation by swallowing smaller amounts of food slowly, and also by putting your utensil down briefly between bites to reduce the speed of your hand-to-mouth conveyor belt.

Hiccupping

You may find yourself hiccupping during your first course. Hiccups signify cramping in your throat muscles from swallowing too forcefully, and often result from swallowing too much, too quickly. When you start to hiccup, you should just relax for a minute or two, and take a few sips of water, until the hiccups eventually stop. If you continue to swallow too enthusiastically, your hiccups will persist.

Nasal regurgitation and hiccupping apply to beans as much as or more than with corn. In the case of nasal regurgitation, you will probably notice it more with smaller bean parts such as broken pieces, split peas, lentils and green peas.

Bowel Movements

Now we need to discuss your bowel movements. Sorry, I know polite people don't usually talk about these things, but seeing it's just the two of us, I won't tell if you don't. Besides, using BM as an abbreviation makes it sound much more acceptable. When most people eat, their food becomes unrecognizable by the time it eventually exits their body as stool. This occurs due to the process of digestion. On The Armonk Diet, your BM experience may change, because undigested food looks the same coming out in your stool as it did when you consumed it. This means that what you see in your toilet bowl will look very much like what you ate not long before. Expect it. Embrace it. Although this phenomenon sometimes arouses concern in those just starting The Armonk Diet, there is no need for anxiety at seeing undigested seeds in your BMs. The more seeds you swallow, and the less second course regular food you eat, the more your stool will resemble the original appearance of your seeds. In addition, the more you restrict your diet to first-course seeds that you swallow whole, the more your BMs will appear unformed and liquidy. You will get used to this with time. At the very least, you can take comfort in seeing proof of the indigestibility of the seeds you swallow, which validates the theory behind The Armonk Diet method.

You will probably start having more BMs than normal, up to several times a day because, when you consume large amounts of food that you don't digest, what goes in must come out. So the number of pounds of indigestible food you swallow every day equals, on average, at least how many pounds of stool you will pass every day. You should mentally prepare yourself for increases in your BM frequency. You might increase your BM frequency from one or less daily to several times daily, each of them larger than what you may previously have thought normal. It definitely helps to have easy access to a toilet.

If you have BMs too frequently or experience diarrhea, try cutting back on your first course seed consumption, or avoiding whole kernel corn in favor of beans, which may bind your stool together a little better than corn. If needed, you can add constipating ingredients to your second course, including the so-called BRAT diet foods (bananas, rice, applesauce, and toast), milk and cheese products, red meat, eggs and unripe bananas. Less healthy foods that can cause constipation, if you want to go in that direction, include fried foods, baked goods high in sugar, and chocolate.

Additional Tips

When You Are Not at Home

When you want to eat a meal or snack during the day and don't have full kitchen facilities available, canned corn remains your best option for appetite control. You can store canned corn just about anywhere, and you can bring it with you when you travel. Although most people prefer swallowing heated corn to room temperature corn when they have the option, you can swallow room-temperature whole kernel corn easily. Just keep a spoon around, and a can opener if your corn does not come in a pop-top can. Room temperature canned corn makes an eminently practical and not-at-all-unpleasant snack or meal substitute. If you also prefer unsalted food, and do not like the excess salt that comes in most cans of corn, you can buy unsalted canned whole kernel corn in most markets. Generic versions of whole kernel corn, such as store brands, do not taste or look much different than the more-expensive national brand-name versions except the name brands may have larger average kernel sizes. But some of the more expensive brands have pull tabs on top to open them. Pull tabs offer convenience, especially if you don't want to keep a can opener handy, such as when you need to eat away from home. Just drain off the liquid and then either swallow the corn spooned straight out of the can, or transfer the corn into a microwave-safe container, and then heat it up. In a microwave, try using the high setting for about 60 seconds per 15-ounce can.

The First Few Weeks

Most dieters experience frequent hunger pangs on a daily basis even before they begin dieting, most likely due to leptin resistance. During your first few weeks of following The Armonk Diet, you should expect to still feel hungry a lot. As your body gets used to its new eating routine, your frequent hunger pangs may slowly abate. However, as you juggle the portions in your first and second courses, you may want to take advantage of the fact that you can alter your meal routine to eliminate most of your second courses completely. You can just substitute as many cans of corn as it takes to fill you up for all your meals, with no weight-control consequences.

Unlike with crash diets, keep in mind that, as you start this new eating regimen, you may not notice any weight loss during the first few days. You will consume so much whole kernel corn that, during the first few days of following this method, and depending on how fast food passes through you, you may temporarily actually gain some weight due to the large quantities of undigested corn taking up space in your intestines. Not to worry, just stick with the plan. Even as you pack your intestines full of corn, your calorie intake will diminish, and the undigested corn does not count against you. You will start to lose weight soon, as you reduce your overall regular food consumption.

If you diligently follow the guidelines for The Armonk Diet, you should expect to lose weight. Once you reach your new set point, if you continue to follow the plan, you should avoid regaining weight. Depending on your activity level and general state of health, you can expect to lose at least small, measurable, amounts of weight from one week to the next. Your daily weight will fluctuate more randomly, due to the fluid retention that occurs from, for instance, consuming salty food, or your bowel movement schedule. So don't worry if, from one day to the next, you do not see your hoped-for loss on the bathroom scale. The weekly trend should show favorable results, at least until you reach your new set point. If you follow The Armonk Diet instructions diligently and cannot lose weight, then you need to take a hard look at how many calories you eat during your second courses each day, and compare them with your body's calorie requirements, which we discussed in Chapter 3. You may need to further increase your first-course seed consumption in order to fill you up enough to reduce your second-course calorie intake. You might also consider consulting with a doctor to look for a possible alternative medical reason to explain your unexpected failure to lose weight.

Reversing the Order of Your Food Courses

Your second course should generally follow your seed-based first course, as you might find it challenging to motivate yourself to swallow seeds after first eating delicious food in the normal way. However, you could choose to switch the order of the courses if you stayed disciplined enough. You would have to set aside, in advance, everything that you wanted to consume in your second course and, once you finished that food, you could continue by swallowing seeds until you felt ready to stop eating completely. But for most of us, let that second course reward you for the diligent seed-swallowing you did in your first course.

How I Follow The Armonk Diet

As you get started following The Armonk Diet, knowing the specific details of my personal routine may offer some guidance as you incorporate this strange new method into your life. Most people will not want to copy my specific meal regimen exactly, so don't feel like you need to, but think of it as a starting point. You will find your own way.

I used to eat multiple meals per day for most of my life. I ate partly out of custom and parental training, but mostly due to frequent hunger cravings. At the beginning of following The Armonk Diet, I needed to swallow two cans of corn in place of every meal or snack, in order to satisfy my hunger enough to lose my desire to eat. I transitioned from eating digestible food to only swallowing corn at all meals except dinner and the vegetable soup I eat to rehydrate after exercising. I designated dinner as my day's eat-for-nutrition meal. And I lost weight.

Eventually, and surprisingly, my hunger pangs diminished, and my need to swallow two cans of corn in place of every meal decreased to one can. In retrospect, my lessened appetite probably reflected my decreased metabolism, the reduced calorie requirements of a thinner body, and no more having to endure carbohydrate withdrawals. Eventually, as long as I kept myself occupied doing just about anything, my corn-swallowing requirement decreased from one can per meal to zero, and I stopped needing to eat between dinners. I make it a game now, to see if I can go a full day without eating anything. If I win the game, I get to eat all I want for my second course at dinner as my prize, along with a sense of accomplishment. Even if I lose the game, and end up snacking on a swallowed can of corn or two, I still get to eat all I want for dinner, and I know the swallowed snacks will not impact my weight. It took about seven months to reach the point of feeling few or no hunger pangs during the day.

My wife claims my mood usually improves substantially after I eat, so I might actually crave food subconsciously all day long. I know I think about food more frequently when no work or activity distracts me, but that does not happen very often since I keep myself pretty busy. On those days when I have time to contemplate hunger for some reason, I might swallow an occasional can of corn or nibble a low-calorie snack such as carrot sticks. But I never lose control of my cravings, since I always have to option to swallow more corn without consequence.

When I first began following The Armonk Diet, I swallowed three cans' (about six cups) worth of corn each day before dinner to test out the concept. As I started to lose weight, I added beans mostly to validate the concept that beans would work as well as corn. Now, my first course starts with swallowing up to 4 pounds of heated soaked uncooked beans. Next I swallow up to another 5 pounds of heated whole kernel corn. I swallowed lesser quantities of corn and beans at the beginning of my diet adventure, but I gradually increased the quantities of both beans and corn over time after I noticed that, when my weight plateaued, I could jump-start further weight loss by increasing my first-course portion size.

Proceeding from beans to corn during my first course, and then to regular food for my second course, gives my meal a nice progression. I prefer beans at the start of my first course, as their firmer texture seems easier to deal with at the start of the meal than later on. Beans' harder consistency makes them slightly more challenging to swallow, especially if you choose uncooked (my preference) or undercooked beans. Whole kernel corn's softer consistency makes it pretty easy to swallow, especially when heated.

I add two teaspoon of extra virgin olive oil (EVOO) to my heated and rinsed-off container of beans, and then shake up the container to distribute the oil evenly, in order to lubricate the beans. This makes the beans much easier to swallow than un-oiled beans. In addition, consuming olive oil provides some health benefits. EVOO may help prevent a type of mental deterioration, known as mild cognitive impairment, seen in early Alzheimer's disease. So you may as well get the potential cognitive benefit of the EVOO and lubricate your beans at the same time. Those two teaspoons of olive oil contain 80 calories, which you might want to know if you count calories. If you only eat beans once a day, I recommend adding two teaspoons of EVOO to the container. Otherwise, one teaspoon per container should suffice, and will cut down on the calories from the oil.

To take you through my current dinner process (you can alter the numbers up or down, depending on your preference), start with an 8-cup container of uncooked beans, prepared as per the instructions in Chapter 10, and then stored in appropriate containers in my refrigerator or freezer. After taking one of the containers out of the refrigerator, loosen the top and heat it on high in your microwave oven for one minute per pound, or four minutes in my case. Drain off the cloudy water left over in the container. Run some hot water into the bean container until it just covers the beans, then reseal it and shake it up a few times. Drain off the liquid and run some more hot water into the container. Repeat until no froth appears on top of the liquid. If you did a good job rinsing when you first prepared your soaked uncooked beans, you won't have to repeat this process more than two or three times.

After draining off the liquid for the last time, add two teaspoons of EVOO, then shake it up and set it aside for your meal. Now open four cans of whole kernel corn (buy a generic brand of sweet unsalted whole kernel golden corn at your local supermarket), pour them into an appropriately sized container, which might include your bean container if you wait until after you finish your beans, and drain off the liquid. Investing in an automatic can opener takes a lot of stress off your hands. Heat it up for about 90 seconds per can, or eight minutes in my case, and drain off any residual liquid. Now bring everything to the table with a soupspoon and a large cup of water. Don't forget to sponge off your counter-top and sink, because bean and corn juices leave a sticky residue.

When you begin your meal, start with beans. You will determine your optimal portion size by trial and error. Spoon as many beans into your mouth as you can comfortably swallow at once. After every few spoonfuls or so, take a sip of water. The water helps fill you up, soothes your throat if bean-swallowing makes your throat crampy, and helps the beans go down if they get stuck. Once you finish the beans, move on to corn, and continue swallowing as many as can fit comfortably in your throat, along with the water sipping. Drink about twelve ounces of water with the beans, and up to another twelve ounces with the corn.

By the time you finish your bean course, your hunger should have mostly dissipated. By the time you finish your corn course, expect to be pretty full. You should no longer *need* to eat, although you may want to. Once you feel full enough, although not necessarily satiated, you have officially completed your first course. Don't fret about swallowing what you would normally consider a ridiculous amount of food. If you swallow too much during your first course and no longer desire to eat, remember to cut back on the quantity for the next time.

Once you finish your first course, you should still have a little room left to eat for nutrition or pleasure. At that point, you know that when you start eating your second course, you will not be driven by hunger. For your second course, start with vegetables. Before I start preparing my portion of corn and beans, I take a one pound bag of frozen broccoli florets out of the freezer, along with a large handful of frozen Brussels sprouts. I arrange them in a large microwave-safe container, and heat them up. Drink more water with your vegetable course. Then I eat a main course of something protein-containing: chicken in a crockpot stew, or a plain chicken breast, or a piece of fish, or combinations of these. You can also munch on raw baby carrots while eating your second course. Once you have eaten enough savory food, proceed to dessert if you need it, which usually means eating fruit. You should avoid prepared desserts such as baked goods or ice cream, if you really want to lose weight. If you can skip dessert, even better; you don't need it. Then, depending on your residual desire to keep eating, you might eat a large bowlful of air-popped popcorn or some kind of healthy cereal such as puffed wheat or rice, oatmeal, or shredded wheat. At this point, usually between 1-2 hours after starting a meal, most mortals would have surrendered to their satiety. But if you have not completely lost the desire to eat yet, you may be falling victim to the eating inertia we discussed earlier.

As you may recall, eating inertia means that once you start eating, absent any good reason to stop, such as feeling uncomfortably full, you will continue to eat. But it's hard to recognize how full you are while you are eating. However, if you consciously choose to take a break from eating and wait for just a little while, your stomach may finally signal your brain that it's okay to stop. With luck, this will happen early, before your stomach becomes physically uncomfortable. By taking a brief break, you may suddenly realize that you have completely lost your desire to eat. So you should take the time and wait a few minutes, toward the end of the meal, to disrupt the inertia of eating. Push away from the table, and walk around for a minute and see if your brain recognizes your stomach's fullness before you get to the point of physical discomfort.

Having said that, if I still feel the need to keep eating, I might eat another bowl of popcorn, some dry plain cereal, a few nuts, or some baby carrots. I do not recommend sweetened or salty cereal or nuts for those actively trying to lose weight, since eating cereal and nuts can lead to excessive calorie intake and slow down your weight loss velocity. However, once you have reached your weight goal and entered the weight-maintenance phase of The Armonk Diet, cereals and nuts can offer a nice alternative to junk food if you still crave a little something more at the end of your meal. We will discuss the health benefits of nuts in Chapter 15. Recommended cereals include plain puffed rice or wheat. I also toast rolled oats myself and eat them plain.

I drink mostly water during my typical day. I drink a cup of instant coffee in the mornings for its health benefits (more details to come in Chapter 15), not specifically for losing weight. I sweeten it with stevia, a no-calorie sweetener, and add a splash of almond milk. Since those who drink two cups of coffee daily fare even better health-wise than those who drink one cup, and since health benefits also accrue to those who drink decaffeinated coffee, my usual morning cup contains one teaspoon each of regular and decaffeinated instant coffee.

My exercise routine, 4 days per week, helps contribute to my weight loss efforts, and keeps me in shape. On the days I exercise, which means jogging on a treadmill, I consume a quart of homemade vegetable soup (you can find the very simple recipe in Chapter 16) to rehydrate after exercising, in addition to the liter of water I drink while jogging. When I started following The Armonk Diet, I sometimes felt hungry even after having the soup, so I would then swallow a can of whole kernel corn, which satisfied me. The soup alone now usually proves sufficient.

As you can tell from the previous paragraphs, as a general rule, I currently only eat one real meal (dinner) every day. I choose not to eat meals except for dinner and the soup I rehydrate with after exercising. That doesn't mean I do not want to eat. Rather, it means that I skip meals because I can. I do not experience desperate or miserable hunger, so I can get away with not eating. However, if I had my druthers, I would eat all the time, which is how I ended up overweight to begin with.

I started out on The Armonk Diet by eating multiple meals and snacks every day. I discovered that losing weight does not depend on how many meals and snacks you eat, but only on swallowing most of your meals in seed form. You can achieve results by just duplicating the methods in this book, regardless of how many times daily you need to eat.

I still consider myself a glutton. I eat, or at least swallow, ridiculous quantities of food during my dinner feast. But, since I swallow most of my meal in seed form and without chewing it, my daily calorie intake stays under control, and my appetite is always satisfied. Also, I do not make an absolute pig of myself during my second course only because my stomach doesn't have room for much more food, due to pigging out during my first course. I also tend to avoid extremely fattening foods such as prepared desserts and sugary or starchy foods as much as possible. I suspect that, if I did not do those things, my weight loss would have proceeded much more slowly.

You can swallow massive, unlimited amounts of corn and beans all day long and get thin and keep it that way. If you need to eat multiple meals per day, go ahead. Just keep an eye on your second course calorie intake, or follow my technique of only eating second course foods once a day. You just need to keep your total daily calorie consumption below your body's maintenance requirements, as we discussed in Chapter 3. If you need massive amounts of food at each feeding, just tilt the distribution of food heavily toward your first course. In case I wasn't clear enough on this point, you can swallow as many cans of corn and containers of beans as it takes to fill you up, all day long, without worrying about how it will impact your weight.

If you suffer from acid reflux or have any other reason not to eat large quantities of food in one sitting the way I do, you should instead eat multiple smaller meals daily. Don't feel compelled to stuff yourself if doing so leads you to experience regurgitation, heartburn or even vomiting due to your fullness. For those with weak stomachs, grazing frequently throughout the day makes more sense than gorging. Just stick to the first course/second course routine with each smaller meal or snack.

Chapter 12: Adding Some Flavor

If you want to try out The Armonk Diet but can't stomach (get it?) the idea of swallowing plain corn and beans, you can tickle your taste buds by adding some low- and no-calorie flavorings to spice things up. Whole kernel corn has a naturally pleasant flavor, which beans lack, so this chapter assumes you want to flavor the beans. However, everything here also potentially applies to corn. Don't bother trying these serving suggestions unless you crave variety in your first courses.

Citrus fruit juices such as lemon and orange juice

A splash of citrus juices can brighten any dish without much of a calorie effect, or you can make a citrus dressing by adding two parts of any citrus fruit juice to one part of olive oil. Olive oil adds 40 calories per teaspoon.

Hot Sauce

Add a few shakes of any of your favorite hot sauces, which often contain few calories, to add some fire.

Fresh Herbs

You can chop up some fresh cilantro and parsley and sprinkle them into your dish, either by themselves, or mixed with olive oil.

Seasoning Blends

All kinds of different seasoning blend flavors populate the aisles of your local market. Most contain a lot of salt. Consider seeking out low-salt versions if you want to reduce your salt intake.

Oregano

We customarily shake oregano onto pizza slices, but you can try it on your first courses, too, or combine it with lemon juice for a Greek-ish flavor.

Indian Spices: Curry, Cumin, and Turmeric

Curry powder contains some or all of the following: coriander, cumin, turmeric, ginger, mustard, fenugreek, pepper, cloves, cardamom, fennel, and cinnamon. You can buy it pre-made or make it yourself, sprinkling it into your first course to create an exotic flavor.

Cumin seeds add a nutty, peppery Middle Eastern flavor. You can add cumin as seeds or in the form of a powder.

Its stunning yellow color makes turmeric visually impressive, and adds a mildly spicy flavor. You can also sauté one part of turmeric with three parts of olive oil and chopped onion, then mix it into your dish.

Fresh Ginger

You can add freshly-grated ginger for a mild spice. Alternative medicine circles often use ginger to treat digestive issues like upset stomach, nausea, and vomiting.

Sautéed Onions and Garlic

Sauté two parts of finely diced onions and one part of garlic with one part of olive oil or cooking spray, then mix it into your dish.

Flavored Vinegars

Try sprinkling some port or champagne vinegar on your beans for a nice change of pace, or just use one of the white, balsamic, cider and/or red wine vinegars already hiding in your cabinets.

Chapter 13: Weight Goals

While determining a goal for how much weight to lose can seem reasonable, you may find setting a general goal of losing weight, period, a less-stressful option. If you decide to set a healthy weight goal, your body mass index (BMI) can help with your planning. You can calculate your BMI by multiplying your weight in pounds by 703 and dividing the result by your height in inches, then dividing again by your height in inches. As an example, if you stand five feet two inches tall (62 inches) and weigh 155 pounds, your BMI equals $703 \times 155/(62 \times 62) = 28.3$. Of course, you can also just go online and enter your height and weight in a BMI calculator, such as one that pops up when you type the words "BMI calculator" into any major web browser's search bar. By convention, a BMI from 25-30 lands you in overweight territory; 30-40 defines obesity; and anything higher than 40 means extremely obese. If your BMI falls under

20, you probably should not try to lose weight so you don't put your health at risk.

Controversy exists over the BMI's usefulness as an indicator of body fat and overall health. Although a "normal" healthy BMI falls in the 18.5-25 range (as defined by the nutrition authorities), a BMI from 25-29.9, which defines you as overweight, may actually lead to better health outcomes. In at least one study, people in the 25-29.9 BMI range had a lower likelihood of dying during the study's observation period than those in the other weight groups. This controversial finding has plenty of detractors, so don't assume it will stand the test of time. But, as a take-home message here, if you want to lose weight, don't convince yourself that you absolutely must get down to the normal BMI range of 18.5-25 unless you want to for reasons of personal preference. At least for health and longevity, you should set a goal of below a BMI of 30.

Chapter 14: Making Healthy Choices

Dieting to lose weight is probably the main reason you bought this book. But don't limit yourself to just one goal of losing weight. Lay the groundwork for attaining the best health possible, as well. That means eating healthier things and living a healthier lifestyle. In this chapter and the next, we will discuss some ways to achieve those goals.

When You Eat

Unlike with some other weight loss plans, The Armonk Diet contains no absolute restrictions on what you can eat. You can eat any regular food you want during the second-course part of your meal. By the time you start eating your second course, hunger should not factor into your eating decisions, hopefully leading to eating less and thus losing weight. However, if you attempt to lose weight while still eating the same amounts of the same junk food you always ate, expect your results to disappoint. If you plan your second courses with some attention to avoiding junk and comfort foods, you will lose weight faster, and your body will thank you by living longer and staying healthier than you otherwise would have.

Treat yourself to a few junk food items if you must, but only after you fill yourself up to the point that you do not feel hungry. Once full, you should stop eating. The sweet and savory deliciousness of junk and comfort foods somehow overrides your feeling of satiety and makes you more likely to continue eating, probably due to those pesky neurotransmitters acting on your brain's pleasure/reward circuits. So you should consider parting ways with your old eating habits, which will free you to reach your full weight loss potential. Save the gluttony for your first course, and swallow all the whole kernel corn and beans you want. Skimp on your second course, limiting your portions to moderate amounts that allow you to stay within a weight-losing calorie range for your best results.

Adhering to a regular eating routine can help make the transition to your new diet almost automatic. Try to eat a consistent diet in a consistent location, preferably at home. Eating at home helps you stay in control of your meals by allowing you to prepare your food yourself as much as possible. But if others prepare your food, don't fret; The Armonk Diet will still work. Just try to avoid meals outside the home, such as in restaurants and cafeterias, if you can. The logistics of trying to follow The Armonk Diet, which relies on large quantities of canned corn and stored beans, outside your home may prove challenging.

Since some people do not have the benefit of regular eating times or locations, it helps to have a fallback option. If you end up frequently eating meals outside of your home because of your hectic life, your travel schedule, vacationing, a social engagement, or for any other reason, you should try not to skip or forget your first course. If you need to skip a first course due to circumstances, you might temporarily backslide on your diet, although you can make up for it pretty quickly if you re-engage as soon as possible. But skipping one first course can lead to skipping more first courses and, soon, you may have inadvertently sabotaged your diet. To prevent this, just try to find a way to incorporate your eating routine into your current situation. You can plan to either bring canned corn with you (pop-top cans of whole kernel corn travel well), or you can purchase some at a local market. Just bring a spoon, and perhaps a can opener. This way, you can at least partly fill yourself up before any meals you eat outside the home, which will hopefully lower the amount of food you otherwise would have eaten.

For Your Heart

If you have a personal or family history of heart disease, the number one killer in the United States, you have the power to do something about it aside from taking powerful drugs. You can reduce your chance of coronary events such as heart attacks, bypass procedures and death from cardiovascular causes by adhering to a favorable lifestyle. If you do stick to a healthy lifestyle, you can expect a nearly 50% reduction in your risk of those coronary events. The four lifestyle factors you need to consider include not currently smoking cigarettes, not being obese (having a BMI less than 30), performing a physical activity at least once a week and having a healthful diet pattern. A healthful diet pattern was defined as doing at least half of the following: eating more fruits, nuts, vegetables, whole grains, fish and dairy products and eating less refined grains, processed meats, unprocessed red meats, sugar-sweetened beverages, trans fat and sodium. We will discuss nutrition more in the next chapter.

If you are at high genetic risk for coronary events because of a family history of heart disease, you may have a greater than 10% risk of having a coronary event in the next 10 years. Following the lifestyle guidelines might decrease that risk to 5%, which should provide you with some motivation to make these changes. Even those at low genetic risk experience similar percentage reductions in coronary events, although their overall number of events is less. This means that lifestyle changes can work better than taking drugs, such as statins, that doctors often prescribe to reduce coronary risk. As an extra benefit, healthy lifestyle changes can also reduce your risk of cancer, the number two killer.

Coming up next is some detailed nutrition advice for achieving optimal health.

Chapter 15: Nutrition Advice

If you take The Armonk Diet to its logical extreme, meaning you consume only first courses and not second courses, you will essentially starve yourself. You will lose weight very rapidly without going hungry, but you will also become malnourished, your body will break down, and you won't keep the weight off for long once you stop dieting. Don't pursue this path without seeking appropriate professional medical advice to prevent complications. The Armonk Diet wants you to lose weight and also to maintain or improve your health. For good health, you need to keep up with your body's nutrition requirements. This chapter focuses on ways to eat healthily. To start, for a healthy diet at the most basic level, you need a combination of the three so-called macronutrients: protein, carbohydrates and fat. In addition, you should pay attention to other dietary factors such as salt, alcohol, caffeine, and fiber, as well as certain supplements.

Protein

Your organs, muscles, skin, hair, nails, bones and certain hormones consist, in large part, of protein. Your body needs protein to build muscle mass and repair damaged cells. An average woman needs 46 grams of protein daily; an average man, 56 grams. A 3 ounce (after cooking) piece of meat such as beef, fish, or chicken, about the size of the palm of your hand, contains 21 grams of protein. Fun fact: although we usually think of meat as purely protein-containing, that's only true for meat's *dry* weight. W*ater* actually comprises most of meat's weight, followed by protein, with a small amount of fat making up most of the rest.

Nine ounces of cooked meat daily will probably satisfy your protein requirement. So you could eat three portions a day of cooked meat, each about the size of your palm. If you don't trust your hand size as a guide, you can use a kitchen scale. If you prefer not to consume so much meat, non-meat alternatives include eggs (a large egg contains approximately 6 grams of protein), yogurt (11 grams in 8 ounces), a cup of whole milk (8 grams), and a cup of quinoa (8 grams). Certain beans also have high protein content. For instance, one cup of soybeans contains 68 grams of protein, and one cup of chickpeas, pinto beans and kidney beans contain around 40 grams. Do the math, and you can mix and match the individual protein amounts in each item to reach the total your body needs, with or without the consumption of meat. Some researchers believe that too much protein can put your health at risk, by making you more prone to kidney disease, diabetes, and cancer, so try to limit your protein intake to 35% of your total calories.

You can avoid less-healthy versions of high-protein foods by trimming excessive fat from your meat and removing the skin from poultry. You should also avoid high-fat processed meats such as bacon, sausages, and cold cuts, as well as organ meats such as liver. Try to avoid egg yolk and whole egg consumption, but feel free to use egg whites and egg substitutes freely, as they contain no cholesterol and minimal fat. If you like regular milk but want a healthier alternative, switch to fat-free or low-fat milk, yogurt and cheese.

Carbohydrates

Most people consume more carbohydrates than fats or proteins. Carbohydrates, also called sugars, serve as your body's main energy source. Dietary carbohydrates include simple sugars as well as the complex carbohydrates known as starch and dietary fiber. During digestion, all carbohydrates except fiber break down into sugars. Sugars and starches occur naturally in many nutritious foods, such as milk, fruits, vegetables, breads, cereals, and grains. Many of these foods contain combinations of all three macronutrients.

In any weight loss program, you should consider eliminating most, but not all, carbohydrates from your diet. Non-starchy vegetables, an exception to that rule, should remain in your diet due to their fiber and vitamin content. Non-starchy vegetables means green vegetables like broccoli, asparagus, peas, leafy greens, and Brussels sprouts, along with other-colored vegetables such as tomatoes, carrots, and cauliflower. You can safely jettison starchy carbohydrates such as potatoes and grains, as well as sugar in any form. People commonly gain weight due to their overconsumption of starchy carbohydrates and sugars.

Fructose, a sugar often found in fruits or added (in the form of high fructose corn syrup) to prepared foods to make them sweeter, gives you another reason to avoid carbohydrates due to its failure to stimulate insulin production in your body. You learned in Chapter 3 that insulin can help reduce your drive to keep eating. But your body only produces insulin after consuming glucose, and not at all after consuming fructose. This explains why some sweet foods containing high levels of fructose, such as fruits and corn syrups, may not effectively reduce hunger despite containing plenty of calories. To reduce your eating drive, you should avoid foods containing large amounts of fructose such as pears and apples. Fruits containing relatively little fructose include apricots, peaches, and plums.

Diabetes is an increasingly common ailment often linked to gaining weight. Successful diabetes management requires optimal blood sugar control. Your best chance at reducing or eliminating your need for diabetes medications relies on eliminating carbohydrates as much as possible. This means increasing your protein and fat consumption by going on a low carbohydrate diet such as the Atkins diet. You can follow such a low-carb diet in conjunction with The Armonk Diet.

Thanks to our friends in the junk food industry, we frequently encounter an evil type of carbohydrate known as added sugars. Added sugars, by definition, do not occur naturally in foods like fruit or milk. Instead, cooks and food scientists add them to foods for extra sweetness during processing or preparation. Your body does not know and cannot tell the difference between naturally-occurring sugars and chemically-identical added sugars. Added sugars, especially in the case of sugar-sweetened beverages, lead to cardiovascular disease. In the United States, non-diet soft drinks such as sodas represent the number one source of added sugars. Other added sugar offenders include sweets, candies, cakes, cookies, and fruit drinks. Added sugar does nothing beneficial for your diet or health. You should drink water instead of sugared sodas and fruit juices if you need something to quench your thirst.

To find out if sugars have been added to your food, just look at the food label ingredient list. Look for terms such as brown sugar, corn sweetener, corn syrup, dextrose, fructose, fruit juice concentrate, glucose, high-fructose corn syrup, honey, invert sugar, lactose, malt syrup, maltose, molasses, raw sugar, sucrose, syrup, and table sugar. If one of these names appears first or second in the ingredient list, or if several of these names appear, that food probably contains excessive sugar. The food industry uses all these different names for sugar in order to confuse consumers into believing that our food choices contain something healthier than just added calories.

Extremely low-calorie sugar substitutes such as saccharin, aspartame, acesulfame potassium, stevia and sucralose offer a sweet taste without the calories. They can help you lose weight if used properly, such as in coffee or tea, which have minimal calories. Most foods that contain sugar substitutes, however, still have calories. Unless you reduce the total number of calories you eat, using sugar substitutes will not help you lose weight.

To summarize, you should avoid excessive carbohydrate consumption by reducing or eliminating most non-vegetable carbohydrates, such as sugar, starchy grains and potatoes. If you need to lose weight, you don't need starches or sugar in your diet. You should avoid white starchy foods such as potatoes, breads, rice, noodles, and anything with added sugar, as well as baked goods. You should eat fresh fruit if you want something for dessert, and avoid high fructose fruits such as apples and pears. You can drink all the water you want, and cut out sugar-sweetened beverages such as sodas and juices.

Fats

Fats do some good things for your body. For instance, they store a lot of the energy that keeps us going, holding on to it until we need it. Fats also supply essential fatty acids, and help you absorb the fat-soluble vitamins A, D, E, and K, as well as carotenoids. Therefore, your meals should contain some fat, just not too much. Of course, if you weigh too much, fat probably comprises most of the excess baggage you need to get rid of. You certainly don't want to add to your fat reservoir by eating excessive amounts of fat, which can lead to weight gain. In addition, you should start thinking about what kinds of fat you eat. The different types of fats you might encounter include saturated fat, unsaturated fat, trans fat, and dietary cholesterol. You should shun trans fats and saturated fats, which increase your risk for a heart problem called coronary artery disease and lead to heart attacks. Although our understanding of trans and saturated fats' evils has led to reduced saturated fat consumption by society, most people still consume too much. Unsaturated fats, in contrast, found mainly in vegetable oils, offer a healthier option.

Saturated Fats

Generally speaking, foods high in saturated fats can raise blood cholesterol, which raises your risk of heart disease. (One interesting exception, stearic acid, found in dark chocolate, does not raise unhealthy cholesterol.) You don't *need* any saturated fats in your diet. Foods to reduce or avoid include high-fat dairy products such as cheese, whole milk, cream, butter, and regular ice cream; fatty meats; the skin and fat of poultry; lard; palm oil; and coconut oil. Diets low in saturated fat help prevent premature death. If you count calories, try to keep your saturated fat intake to less than 7% of your daily calories, which translates to 16 grams of saturated fat daily on a 2000 calories per day diet.

Cholesterol

Fact: high LDL (low density lipoprotein, or "bad" cholesterol) levels correlate with increased risk of heart disease. Another fact: foods high in cholesterol can raise blood cholesterol for some individuals. Therefore, at least *some* people should refrain from consuming large amounts of cholesterol. Unfortunately, no simple test can tell how sensitive you are to dietary cholesterol. Therefore, out of caution, you should try not to over-indulge in dietary cholesterol, and so avoid egg yolks, shellfish, liver and other organ meats, and dairy fats.

Trans Fats

Foods high in trans fats (also called trans fatty acids) raise your health risk the most of all the fats. You should avoid foods containing trans fats completely. Unfortunately, foods high in trans fats often taste the best. High trans fat foods include fried foods and fast foods, such as chips, cookies, crackers, doughnuts, pastries, pie crust, and pizza. High trans fat foods contain partially hydrogenated vegetable oils in the ingredient list, especially in many hard margarines and shortenings. Trans fats raise LDL blood cholesterol, and increase your risk of heart disease and diabetes. If you cannot eliminate your exposure to trans fats, at least try to limit the total to less than 1% of your total calories, or 2 grams on a 2000 calorie diet. Interestingly, no thanks to our convoluted food labeling laws, your food can contain trans fats even when the food nutrition label says it does not, because the nutrition labeling rule states that any amount under 0.5 grams/serving counts as 0 grams. So, many unhealthy prepared foods have labels that fail to make clear their health risk. Our nutrition labels should indicate the presence of even small amounts of trans fats.

Unsaturated Fats

Unsaturated fats (and oils) do not raise blood cholesterol and allow for a healthy fat option. You can find unsaturated fats, in *monounsaturated* or *polyunsaturated* form, in most nuts, olives, avocados, vegetable oils, and fatty fish such as salmon. Monounsaturated fats include canola, olive, peanut and sunflower oils; polyunsaturated fats include corn oil, cottonseed oil, soybean oil, and many kinds of nuts. Eating an ounce of nuts daily reduces your risk of coronary artery disease, respiratory diseases, diabetes and cancer. Some fish, such as salmon, tuna, and mackerel, also contain omega-3 fatty acids, another type of unsaturated fat that may protect against heart disease. You can feel good about eating moderate amounts of food high in unsaturated fats, taking care to avoid excess calories. Substituting unsaturated for saturated fats lowers your risk of heart disease.

For optimal health, try to keep your total fat intake to 35% or less of your total calories, from foods such as fish, nuts, and vegetable oils, and avoid trans fats completely. Cook with vegetable oils rather than solid fats such as lard. Reduce calories by decreasing the amount of butter or oil you use in cooking and at the table. When choosing prepared foods, look for those foods lowest in saturated fat and cholesterol.

Salt

Table salt, chemically known as sodium chloride, makes food taste better. Our parents usually get us hooked on salt as children. Parents tend to salt many naturally bland or bitter foods, such as broccoli and cauliflower, as a way to introduce them into children's diets. In theory, once you get used to eating the salted version of a food, your maturing palate can eventually graduate to the unsalted version, but not everyone successfully makes that transition.

Although some of us pour salt directly onto our food from a salt shaker, most of our salt comes from the processed/prepackaged foods we buy. A healthy adult requires less than 500 milligrams of table salt (¼ teaspoon) daily, an amount that many of us exceed several-fold. Since salt makes food taste more appealing, it makes you want to eat more food, compared with unsalted food. Salt also makes you thirsty, so you drink and retain more fluids. These factors both lead to weight gain. Therefore, reducing or eliminating salt can help you lose weight. If you change to a no-added-salt diet, you may lose a couple of pounds of water weight within just a few days, even *without* reducing your calorie intake. One gram of salt will cause you to retain more than 1 ½ pounds of water, which will stay in your body for about three days before you eliminate that extra salt and fluid by urination. So don't assume that you suddenly gained a lot of extra weight after a salty meal or snack, because it may just be water weight from the salt.

From a weight loss perspective, cutting out salt seems like a no-brainer due to its short term benefit. From a health perspective, however, things get more confusing. Most people do not need to limit their salt consumption for health reasons, and some evidence even suggests that too little salt consumption can cause health problems.

Excessive salt consumption has some known negative health consequences. For instance, high salt intake increases the amount of calcium excreted in your urine, which increases your risk of osteoporosis and bone fractures. If you have Meniere's disease, an uncommon inner ear problem, consuming salt can provoke an attack of vertigo. More familiar to most of us, salt consumption may affect your heart. Not-so-fun fact: about one in three American adults has high blood pressure. You can reduce your chances of developing high blood pressure by consuming less salt. If you already have high blood pressure, however, consuming greater amounts of salt raises your risk of heart attacks, strokes, and death. So some of us need to worry about high salt intake, although most of us do not. You should discuss your salt intake with your doctor at your next visit.

If you want to reduce your salt intake for either health or weight control reasons, start by cutting back on added salt and salty foods and seasonings. Unsalted food may seem less appealing for a week or two while you adjust to the natural flavors of your food. Your preference for salt may decrease if you lower your sodium intake gradually, such as by adding smaller amounts of salt or salty seasonings to your food over a period of time. As a bonus, if you stick to a low-salt lifestyle, you might gain a greater appreciation for the subtle tastes of food in its natural, unaltered state. Many who transition to a low- or no-salt diet subsequently find salty food unappetizing.

Not everyone who wants to reduce their salt consumption should stop suddenly. If you exercise vigorously, you should gradually decrease the amount of salt you consume, rather than going cold turkey. When you exercise heavily or in high heat, you might lose dangerous amounts of sodium via sweating and experience dehydration if you abruptly remove salt from your diet.

To decrease your salt intake, choose mostly plain water, which usually contains minimal salt, to drink. At home, add smaller amounts of salt to your usual recipes, or no salt at all. Many recipes that call for salt taste perfectly delicious if prepared unsalted. Use other spices and herbs, rather than salt, if you want to flavor your food (refer back to Chapter 12 for suggestions). Avoid salty condiments such as ketchup, mustard, olives, pickles, and soy sauce. Put your salt shaker away.

At the store, choose fresh fruits, meats and vegetables and avoid canned and processed versions. Read the food label to compare the amount of sodium in processed foods such as breads, cereals, cheese, frozen dinners, packaged mixes, salad dressings, sauces, and soups. Look for "low sodium" on labels.

When eating out, order grilled or roasted entrees without sauces, steamed vegetables, and salad with oil and vinegar. Avoid salty dishes such as batter-fried foods, stews, and sauced pasta. Tell the waiter you want no salt added to your food.

Alcohol

Alcohol offers at least one health benefit in addition to its mind-altering qualities. Drinking in moderation (no more than one drink per day for women and two drinks for men) may lower your risk for coronary artery disease, mainly among men over age 45 and women over age 55. If you drink alcohol mainly to reduce your heart disease risk, however, you should know that you can do other things to reduce your risk just as much or more, including eating a healthy diet, getting physical activity, stopping smoking, and maintaining a healthy weight.

Alcohol has a number of drawbacks. Alcoholic beverages supply calories but little nutrition, and so lead to gaining weight. Excess alcohol impairs judgment and can lead to addiction. Alcohol raises your risk of developing cancer, high blood pressure, stroke, malnutrition, and damaged organs such as liver, pancreas, brain and heart. Alcohol leads to violence, suicide, motor vehicle accidents, other kinds of injuries, and social and psychological problems. If a woman drinks alcohol during pregnancy, her baby may have birth defects.

Alcohol is best enjoyed in moderation. You should not drink alcohol during childhood, pregnancy, when driving or operating machinery, and if taking prescription or over-the-counter medications that can interact with alcohol.

Coffee and Tea

Drinking a cup or two of coffee or black or green tea every day, if you can tolerate it, provides some potentially compelling health benefits, but probably won't help you lose weight. Coffee, for instance, may protect against a number of ailments, such as adult-onset diabetes, Parkinson's disease, multiple sclerosis, liver disease, liver and colorectal cancer, and heart failure, and may prevent premature death. Tea may reduce your risk of stroke and heart disease, liver disease and cancer, depression, and diabetes. You should limit yourself to moderate amounts of coffee and tea due to their stimulant effects, which can interrupt sleep. The downsides of drinking coffee include risks of acid reflux, anxiety, depression, reducing a woman's chances of becoming pregnant, and disrupting your body's internal clock. You should not drink coffee late in the day, or if you have high blood pressure. If you did not previously drink coffee or tea, and have no reason why you can't, you might consider starting by drinking a cup or two of coffee in the mornings, sweetened with an artificial sweetener such as stevia, and maybe with a splash of milk to reduce the acidity.

Advice for Food Prepared in Restaurants

Many restaurants do not share nutrition information about their menu options. As a general rule, weight loss efforts suffer in restaurants due to increasingly large portion sizes; excessive use of butter, salt, and sugar to increase food's appeal; your misplaced inclination not to waste food; and the potential social embarrassment of stopping eating before everyone else at your table. But you *can* request no salt and butter, and seek out healthier menu selections. You should look for fish or lean meats, and avoid ground meat, fatty processed meats, marbled steaks, and cheese. Try to limit your intake of creamy sauces, and choose fruits for dessert.

Additional Nutrition and Supplement Advice

Vitamins and Minerals

Most Americans consume plenty of vitamins and minerals in the food they eat. You do not need vitamin supplements unless a doctor has diagnosed you with a vitamin deficiency. However, if you do not eat a well-rounded diet, for instance because you choose to follow a very low calorie diet, you should take a multivitamin every day, as a precaution against becoming vitamin deficient.

Thinning bones, called osteopenia or osteoporosis (osteoporosis is the more severe version), can occur as you age. Usually diagnosed with x-rays of your bones, osteoporosis raises your risk of bone fractures, especially in women. You can help counteract this by consuming enough calcium from food. Calcium helps build strong bones. Foods high in calcium include dark leafy greens, cheese, low-fat milk and yogurt, bok choy, fortified tofu, okra, broccoli, green beans, almonds, and fish canned with their bones. You might consider taking a calcium supplement if you do not obtain enough calcium from food. Most adults need 1000-1200 mg of calcium daily, along with vitamin D3 (600 international units), which helps your body absorb the calcium. You can find this combination inexpensively in 2 tablets daily of Kirkland Signature Calcium 600 mg + D3, or other brands. Calcium can also cause side effects such as raising your risk of kidney stones, constipation, heart attacks, and gastrointestinal problems. But if you passed age 50, an age when your risk of bone fractures starts going up, the benefits may outweigh the risks. You should discuss this with your doctor.

Herbal Supplements

Most herbal supplements have no proven benefit for human health. Often prescribed by practitioners of oriental medicine, some herbs can cause damage. You should avoid them unless your doctor makes a medical recommendation to take them. Most herbal supplements, derived from plants, contain many different compounds. Some of the compounds may have desired therapeutic effects, but other compounds in the

150

same herb may have toxic effects, despite herbs' "natural" origin. "Natural" does not always equal "safe." In addition, the potency of different batches of herbs can vary, making it hard to know how much to take. If your doctor suggests treatment with herbs, you should ask if there is alternative available as a prescription medication, and let your doctor explain why the herb is a better choice for you.

Fiber

Fiber can help you feel full, and can therefore assist in any effort to lose weight. Your body cannot digest fiber in the same way that it cannot digest the seeds you swallow during your first course, so it does not add calories to your diet. Fiber comes in two types: soluble, meaning dissolvable in water; and insoluble, which doesn't dissolve in water. Soluble fiber, when it dissolves, forms a gel, and provides health benefits such as lowering blood cholesterol and glucose levels. Insoluble fiber promotes stool transit through your digestive system and increases stool bulk, which can benefit those who struggle with constipation or irregular stools. You can find soluble fiber in apples, barley, beans, carrots, citrus fruits, oats, and peas, among other things. Good sources of insoluble fiber include whole grains, beans, nuts, vegetables such as broccoli, and fruits with their skins. Healthy adults need between 20-40 grams of total fiber daily. As points of reference, a 15 ounce can of whole kernel corn contains about 7 grams of fiber, and a similarly-sized can of red kidney beans contains about 28 grams of fiber.

Aspirin

Aspirin, the common name for acetylsalicylic acid, relieves pain and fever and reduces blood clotting. In the case of a heart attack, aspirin can literally save your life. It may prevent certain types of cancers as well. Many doctors recommend aspirin in an 80 mg/day dose, called baby aspirin, in order to keep blood from clotting in patients at high risk for blood clot-induced heart attacks and strokes. However, due to its blood-thinning properties, aspirin can cause a nosebleed or heavy menstrual periods, can lead to prolonged bleeding if you accidentally cut yourself, and may result in larger-than-usual bruises. The older you get, the more likely your physician will recommend taking a daily baby aspirin in order to reduce your risk of heart attacks and strokes. You should not take aspirin regularly unless your doctor believes that the benefits outweigh the disadvantages.

Chapter 16: Some Simple Home Meal Ideas

Following The Armonk Diet does not require making any special dietary sacrifices, although it helps to prepare your own food yourself in order to avoid unhealthy ingredients. Plus, controlling your own food preparation means no inadvertent consumption of ingredients you might prefer to avoid. Anyone with a modicum of experience cooking can find numerous healthy recipes from outside sources or create their own dishes by creatively heeding the nutrition advice from the previous chapter. If you consider yourself proficient in the kitchen, you should go ahead and follow your dietary muse with my best wishes, and feel free to ignore the rudimentary recipes in this chapter. The ridiculously simple recipes here will not particularly appeal to people who already know how to cook. If, on the other hand, you don't cook much and need some advice on how to get started cooking simple and healthy food for yourself, you have come to the right chapter. These recipes can serve as a starting point for people who have no background in food preparation and need some meal ideas.

Unfortunately, my home, like many others, suffers from a dearth of available meal preparation time, and possibly also from a little bit of laziness and a lack of enthusiasm about cooking. So, we turn to slow cookers to make many of the various recipes through which we sporadically rotate. Slow cookers (such as the Crock Pot brand, and others) allow us to put a bunch of ingredients in a pot, turn it on, leave home for the day, and have a meal ready when we get home. You can substitute any ingredients you like for the ingredients in these recipes, and you can modify these recipes endlessly.

If you prefer to rely on recipes that you already know and love, you can also use *them*, but cut out the oil, butter, sugar, and salt. This will allow you some of the familiarity of your favorite foods, while removing most of the unhealthy ingredients.

The recipes that we use consist primarily of wholesome ingredients. If you want extra salt, you can add it. If your palate requires extra spice, toss it in. Chicken forms the protein basis of our slow cooker meals. Don't like chicken? Use any other form of protein you like: other meats, eggs, and beans, for instance. We cook our dishes for 6.5 hours in a slow cooker on high heat, which makes the chicken soft and easy to break apart. If you prefer a firmer consistency for your chicken or vegetables, try cooking for 5.5 hours and/or on low heat. We add frozen vegetables, rather than fresh, solely for the time-saving convenience. Feel free to use fresh vegetables if you prefer them. At the end, you will have a large pot full of food that can last for several meals, and cleanup involves just removing a plastic liner from the cooker, and washing the stoneware with soap and water.

Without further ado, here are some simple recipes you can try.

Hominy Chicken

Hominy is a variation of corn that I have considered a special treat since childhood. Adding hominy to a slow-cooked chicken stew makes the stew deliciously memorable.

Chicken breasts, 2 pounds
Dried oregano, 1 tbsp at the start, and reserve another 1 tsp for the end
Cumin, 2.5 tbsp at the start, and reserve another 1 tsp at the end
Frozen cauliflower, 1 pound
Frozen broccoli, ½ pound
Frozen sliced peppers, ½ pound
Garlic, crushed or diced from a jar, 3 tsp
Sliced jalapeno peppers from a jar, 3 tbsp
Unsalted chicken broth, 2 cups
Hominy, 2 15-oz cans, rinsed well and drained
Cornmeal, 2 tbsp if desired

Place a liner in your slow cooker and spray the liner with a nonstick cooking spray (such as Pam). Place a layer of chicken breasts (trimmed of visible gristle and fat) on the bottom of your slow cooker. Shake the oregano and cumin over the chicken liberally. Add the frozen cauliflower and broccoli. On top of that, add the frozen sliced peppers. Add garlic (crushed or diced). Add sliced jalapeno peppers, scattered on top. Add 2 cups of unsalted chicken broth. Cook, covered, on high for 6.5 hours. When done, stir well to break up the chicken into chunk sizes that you prefer. Add the hominy. Shake in another tsp each of cumin and oregano. Add the cornmeal if you prefer a thicker consistency of the liquid. Stir again and then cook for 15 minutes on high to blend and heat through.

Betsy's Chicken Stew

This straightforward chicken stew provides days' worth of hearty food.

Chicken breasts, 2 pounds
Frozen chopped onions, ¼ cup or onion powder, ½ tsp
Garlic, crushed or minced, 1 tsp or garlic powder, 1 tsp
Salt and pepper to taste
Low salt cream of mushroom soup (such as Campbell's), 10-oz can
Low salt cream of chicken soup, 10-oz can
Frozen broccoli, 1 pound
Frozen cauliflower, 1 pound
Frozen mixed vegetables, 1 pound or more
Low salt chicken broth, 2 cups

Place a liner in your slow cooker and spray the liner with a nonstick cooking spray (such as Pam). Place a layer of chicken breasts (trimmed of visible gristle and fat) on the bottom of your slow cooker. Cover the chicken with the onions and garlic. Add salt and pepper here, if desired. Add ½ can of the cream of mushroom soup. Spread it evenly over the chicken (do not dilute with liquid). Add the vegetables, filling your slow cooker almost to the top. While you add the vegetables, add the rest of the can of mushroom soup in the middle of the vegetables. Add the cream of chicken soup (not diluted) atop the vegetables, spread out evenly. Add the chicken broth. Cook, covered, on high for 6.5 hours. When done, stir well to break up the chicken into chunk sizes that you prefer.

Indian-inspired Chicken Stew

I love everything about Indian spices: their colors, taste, and aroma. Adding Indian spices to a basic chicken stew recipe brings a taste of the exotic home.

Chicken breasts, 2 pounds
Turmeric, 1 tsp
Cinnamon, ½ tsp
Garam masala powder, 1 tsp
Cardamom powder, 1 tsp
Ginger, fresh or powdered, ½ tsp
Red chili powder, ½ tsp
Black pepper, ½ tsp
Bay leaves, dry, two
Frozen onion, ¼ cup, or dried powdered onion, ½ tsp
Crushed tomatoes, 32 ounce can (optional, if you like tomatoes)
Fresh or frozen vegetables of your choice, which should include 1 pound of chopped cauliflower for a creamy texture. We also add 1 pound of broccoli florets, and 1-2 pounds of frozen mixed vegetables
Chicken broth, low salt, 2 cups
Coconut milk, one 14-16 oz can of light or regular, if desired

Place a liner in your slow cooker and spray the liner with a nonstick cooking spray (such as Pam). Place a layer of chicken breasts (trimmed of visible gristle and fat) on the bottom of your slow cooker. Pour the spices directly on top of the chicken. Pour the onion over the spices, and add the bay leaves. Pour the tomatoes in next, if you use them. Add the frozen cauliflower and broccoli, then the frozen mixed vegetables. Pour in the chicken broth. Cook 5.5-6.5 hours on high. Remove the bay leaves. If desired, add the can of coconut milk. When done, stir well to break up the chicken into chunk sizes that you prefer.

Vegetable Soup

    I eat this very low-salt concoction to help me rehydrate after vigorous exercise. It helps replace some of the fluid lost. If you want saltier soup, you can change the low-salt chicken broth to regular, or to beef broth, which has even more salt. I use frozen vegetables, mostly for the convenience. Fresh vegetables make an excellent substitute.

Frozen chopped onions, 12 oz
Frozen cauliflower, 1 pound
Frozen sliced carrots, 1 pound
Frozen chopped spinach, or any other leafy green vegetable, such as kale. You could also try cut okra.
Low-salt chicken broth, 1-2 cups
Salt, pepper, or additional herbs/spices to taste

Put a large pot on the stove (I use a 6 quart pot), and turn the heat to high. Pour the onions into the pot. As the pot heats up, stir the onions to sauté them if you prefer non-crunchy onions. Add the sliced carrots, cauliflower, and chopped spinach. Add any other vegetables you want. Fill the pot about 2/3 full with frozen vegetables. Add 1-2 cups of low salt chicken broth. Use regular chicken or beef broth if you want more salt. Fill the rest of the pot with water, until the soup reaches 1 inch below the rim. Add any spices you like, such as pepper or extra salt. I keep my version plain. Let the water boil, and then reduce the heat to simmer, and let it simmer for about an hour, less if you like your vegetables firmer. If it boils or simmers for so long that the water level lowers, add more water to the pot at the end. Once the soup cools, separate into portions. I recommend filling one-quart containers about 2/3 of the way to the top before refrigeration, and usually get about 7 servings from a pot. When ready to reheat the soup, add water to fill a quart container nearly to the top. In the microwave, loosen the lid on the container, and heat on high for 5 minutes.

Following these recipes can help you attain good health. However, don't feel compelled to do so in order for The Armonk Diet to work. Ultimately, it doesn't matter what you eat as long as you diligently follow the method. Once you fill yourself up with food that doesn't count against your weight, you can eat anything you want, within reason. You just need to recognize that eating anything you want does not give you a license to overdo your second course. Remember, you can lose one pound a week by reducing your calorie intake to 500 calories per day less than your body's maintenance requirement. If your body needs 2000 calories per day to maintain its present weight and you want to lose one pound per week, you need to restrict your calories to 1500 per day. Although your body will appreciate the health benefits of you obeying the nutrition suggestions above, you can still, for example, eat two McDonald's Big Macs and an order of fries every day, which totals less than 1500 calories, along with all the whole kernel corn and beans you can swallow, and you will still lose weight as long as you don't consume any other digestible foods. I suspect that the health benefits of losing weight probably offset the detrimental health effects of eating junk food in reasonable quantities. Nevertheless, I recommend healthier eating choices overall. Look at your weight loss attempt as an opportunity to start a new lifestyle built around healthy meal choices.

Chapter 17: Endnotes

So there you have it: a radical new weight loss diet plan that lets you stuff your face and lose weight while you do it. Hopefully, I helped you understand a little bit about why we gain weight and why conventional treatments don't work very well for most people. With any luck, you can benefit from my experience in following this method to slim down. You have the opportunity to put this plan into practice for yourself now, along with some helpful suggestions about what to eat and do for optimal health. I hope that the message in this book resonates with you and motivates you to give The Armonk Diet a try, and that you are able to achieve the weight loss you desire and deserve.

If you have any comments about this book, including suggestions on how to improve it, please email me at info@armonkdiet.com. By following The Armonk Diet, I successfully fulfilled by weight loss goal, and then some. With just a little effort, you can, too. I wish you the best of luck in reaching your own weight loss goal. Let me know how The Armonk Diet works out for you.

Made in the USA
Middletown, DE
17 June 2023

32289796R00096

16: WALDKAUZ-BALZ - WALTER TILGNER, GERMANY

Tawny Owl (*Strix aluco*)

Buchenaltholz on the Bodanrück peninsula near Allensbach (Baden-Württemberg / Germany) 22nd November 2011. Mikrophone: TELINGA CLIP-ONS. Recorder: OLYMPUS LS-11. Extract from a long-term recording. Processed with ADOBE AUDITION.

www.natur-tilgner.de

17: WHAT BIRDS SING - DAVID ROTHENBERG, UNITED STATES OF AMERICA

Superb starling (*Lamprotornis superbus*), white-rumped shama (*Copsychus malabaricus*), Bali Mynah (*Leucopsar rothschildi*)

Recorded at the National Aviary, Pittsburgh, 2004.
David Rothenberg, soprano saxophone Michael Pestel, flute
© *Mysterious Mountain Music (BMI).*

http://davidrothenberg.wordpress.com

Animal Music
Compiled by Lasse-Marc Riek / Gruenrekorder.
Mastered by Dirk Fischer at EvenFlow studios Berlin.
Field Recording Series by Gruenrekorder
Gruenrekorder / Germany / 2015
Gruen 121 / LC 0